Spectacular Superfoods

CHANGE YOUR DIET, CHANGE YOUR LIFE

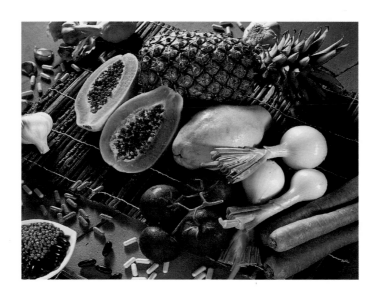

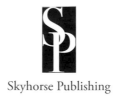

Skyhorse Publishing

Thanks to:

Mercedes Blasco, Montse Bradford, Iona Purtí, Dr. Barnet Meltzer, Dr. Frederic Viñas, Dr. Ramón Roselló, Dr. Miquel Pros Casas, Dr. Pedro Ródenas, Dr. Bernard Jensen, Francesc Fossas (dietitian), Julio Peradejordi, and Vicky Egson.

Library of Congress Cataloging-in-Publication Data is available on file.

Photography: Becky Lawton, Montañés & Gebia, archivo Océano Ámbar, Cristina Reche, Mar Pons, Rosa Castells-CCL, Visió de Futur, Photoalto, Cordon Press, Stock Photos.

Food styling: Menchu Bou, Adriana Ortemberg, Susana Britez, Mercè Esteve.
Illustrations: Emma Schmidt

Cover design by Eric Kang

Print ISBN: 978-1-5107-0551-7
Ebook ISBN: 978-1-5107-0556-2

Printed in China

Spectacular Superfoods

ADRIANA ORTEMBERG

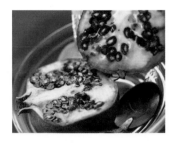

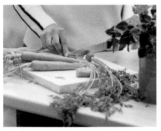

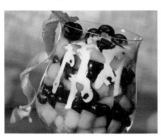

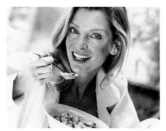

"Eat well, feel well" 10

A balanced diet 13
Food categories
Daily dietary needs
Top ten foods for a well-balanced diet
Superfoods to improve your sex life

Age and food 41
The first months
After twelve months
After age five
Adolescence
Adulthood
Old age

Superfoods 51
What to eat?
Choosing the best options
Types of additives
Nutraceuticals
Frozen food
GMOs
Irradiated food
Organic food
Superfoods
Food for hormonal problems
Food to prevent premature aging
Food to strengthen the joints
Food for healthy bones
Food for a healthy heart

Food combinations 101
How to combine food
Food compatibility charts
Eat everything . . . but not all at once (food
    and weight control)
Living without heartburn: The delicate
    balance between enzymes

Utensils and cooking techniques 113
Food preservation
Preparing food
Cooking utensils

Recipes 127
Assorted salads
Vegetable broth: A medicinal food
Hot and cold soups
Rice
Potatoes
Pasta
Vegetables
Pizzas and quiches
Crêpes and potato patties
Oriental dishes
Mushrooms and special dishes
Desserts
Juices and drinks
Guide to eating well when you are short on
    time
The best and worst diets
Glossary

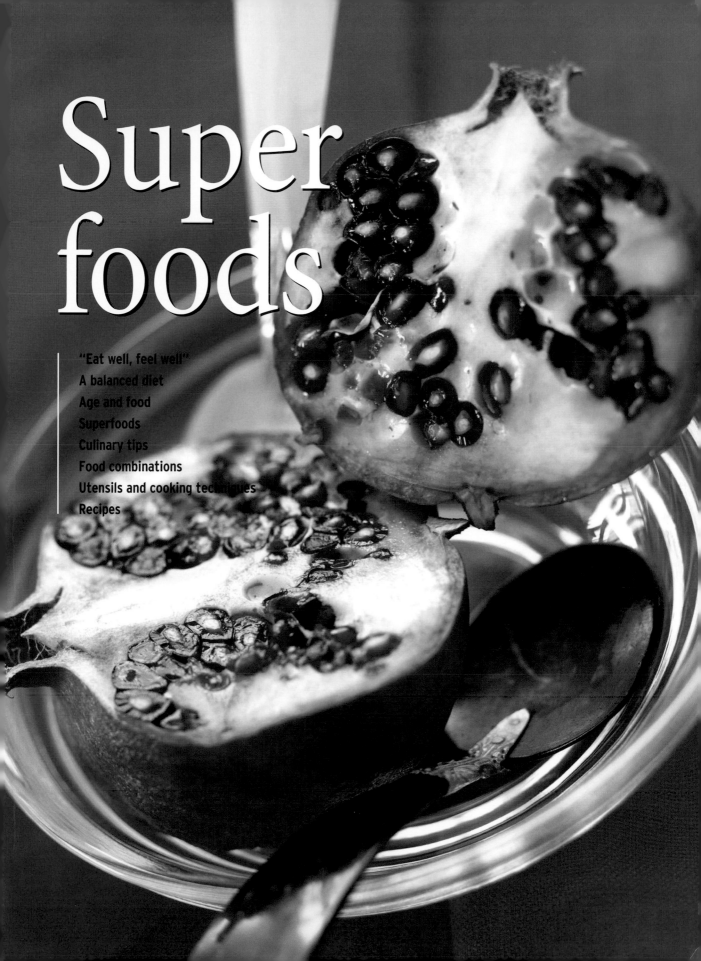

Super foods

"Eat well, feel well"
A balanced diet
Age and food
Superfoods
Culinary tips
Food combinations
Utensils and cooking techniques
Recipes

Editor's note: "Eat well, feel well"

At the end of the day you may feel exhausted, irritable, nervous, or with a mixture of emotions otherwise known as stress. There is a close relationship between what we eat and our emotional, physical and psychological health. Yogis usually remember that happiness depends on adequate **breathing**, **food**, and **activity**, coupled with a positive **mental attitude**.

This is the purpose of this book: to promote wellness through small and simple changes that are very powerful for fostering better health without giving up tasty food. Its aim is to help you become more familiarized with a range of "preferable" foods to help you enjoy optimal health. After many years of experience in the publication of two well-known magazines dedicated to the health and welfare of the body and mind, we have tried to summarize this work, by updating our basic knowledge of nutrition and health and using one of life's most delicious pleasures: good food and its unparalleled range of flavors.

Pear and almond drink.

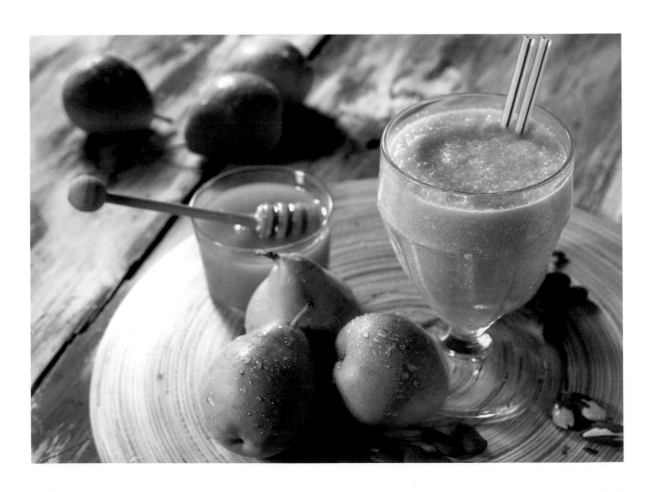

We also include the latest findings in nutrition and dietetics; for instance, the new generation of nutritional supplements, and findings on the benefits of antioxidant foods that are important to help prevent disease and slow aging. Antioxidants? Sure: whose mouth doesn't water when they think of the delicious taste of strawberries (a well-known antioxidant) harvested in season?

Spectacular Superfoods is part of and complements a series of books on food, dietetics, and cooking that are listed in the last pages. We have tried to avoid technicalities as well as food items that are rare or difficult to find. Our recommendations include foods that are easy to find in stores. We also make references for further reading on "superfoods." We will review the virtues and properties of humble vegetables as well as "nutraceuticals," the latest nutritional supplements to hit the market.

We also include tips for preparing and cooking food, and how to best mix ingredients in order to enhance their benefits.

In general, how our emotions and moods are affected by what we eat (and how we eat) is something known and accepted by specialists. Within this same publishing house, you will find *Alimentación equilibrada,* by Barnet Meltzer, and *Alquimia en la cocina,* by Montse Bradford; both of which are largely focused on this important subject that affects our lives much more than it seems.

Finally, there is a significant section of practical recipes for you to use and take advantage of these superfoods. Remember, as the yogis like to say: "An ounce of practice is better than a ton of theory."

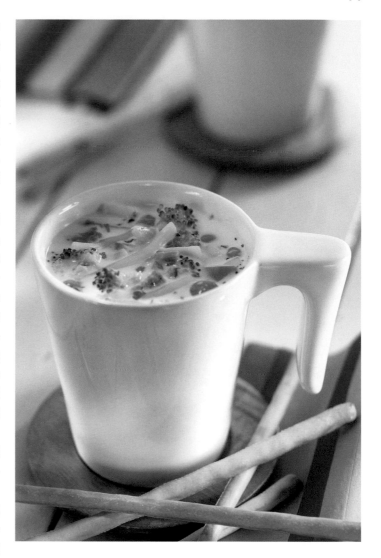

So, we hope that this summary of what you can do to eat better and healthier will be as useful to you as it was exciting for us to edit.

Cream of spring vegetables.

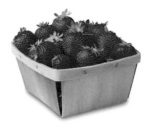

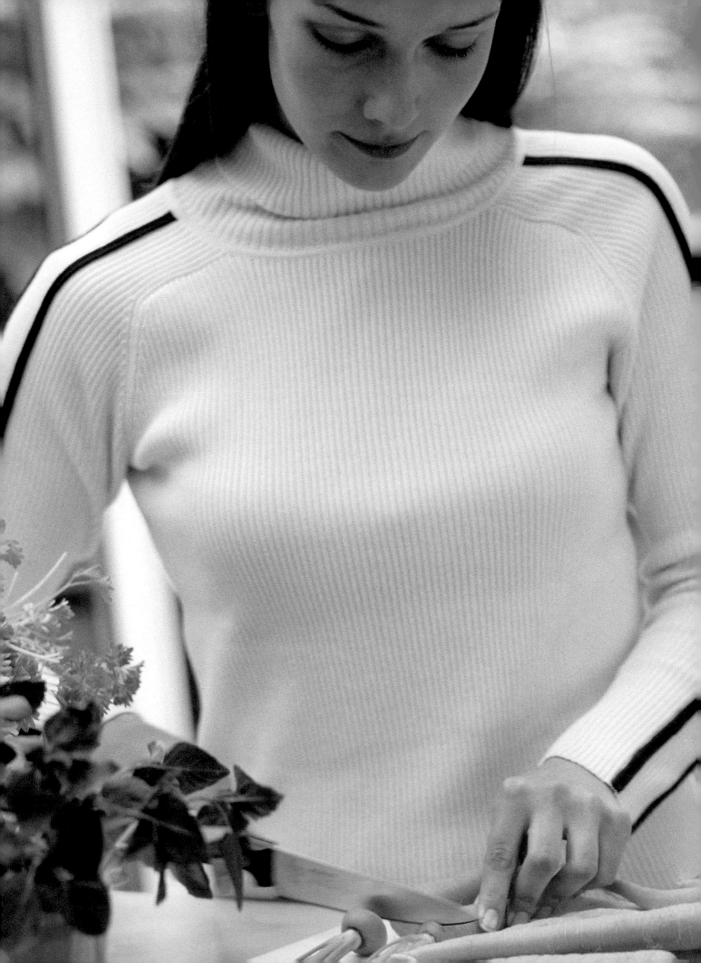

A balanced diet

1 Food categories
Daily dietary needs
Top ten foods for a well-balanced diet
Superfoods to improve your sex life

The foods we eat every day are more than just flavors and aromas that momentarily delight us. So we should try to make them as healthy as possible, and have them meet our daily energy needs. The secret to having a healthy diet is knowing the nutritional properties of each food, as well as ensuring that we have variety, good combinations, and reasonable proportions.

Except for water, the nutrients that our bodies require are not isolated, instead they are part of other substances: food. This means that the only way to get them is by eating foods that contain a certain amount of said nutrients. We will review this information through traditional food classification, and using several interesting charts to help us choose our foods.

When choosing what and how we eat, we all choose to follow certain dietary guidelines.

EATING WELL OR DIETING?

Many people believe that eating well is the same as "dieting": guidelines that are prescribed for weight loss or curing a disease. This is not entirely wrong, but "diet" is a much broader concept: it refers to what we eat and how we eat.

Dieting means following a particular food outline depending on certain circumstances, such as individual factors (age and health, energy needs, tastes, etc.) and external reasons (geographic, economic, seasonal, etc.). Oftentimes, we suffer disorders that can be cured or mitigated simply through proper nutrition. Sometimes, a particular situation (such as overworking), condition (pregnancy, lactation, etc.), or age determine different nutritional requirements. Let's examine this a little more closely.

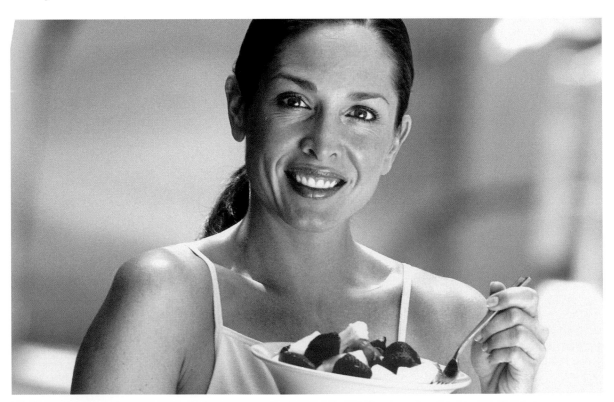

Food Categories

We normally classify foods based on their nutritional content. Although there is no universal classification accepted by all dietitians, since some prefer to group them according to their origin (plant or animal) or their role in the body, the most common consists of six groups.

GRAINS AND STARCH

Foods in this group (wheat, rice, corn, barley) are both raw and in the form of flour. They provide protein, vitamins (especially B group), and carbohydrates, one of the main sources of energy in the body. They have considerable caloric value and, except for the tubers (potatoes, sweet potatoes, etc.), hardly contain water.

• **Rice.** It has much less fat than wheat. It has hypotensive properties and low sodium and potassium, which makes it particularly good for treating heart and kidney disorders. It is not astringent.

• **Oats.** Grain from the northernmost regions. It is highly recommended for its energizing and stimulating capacity, as its nutritional elements act on the thyroid gland. It is also diuretic and hypoglycemic, so it is highly recommended for diabetics.

• **Barley.** It is the grain with the highest amount of sugars (hence its use in alcoholic beverages) and has soothing and refreshing properties. When ingested as sprouted grains, it synthesizes diastase, which aids in the digestion of starches.

• **Rye.** Although it has less gluten than wheat and virtually no vitamin B3 (PP), it increases blood flow, so when eaten frequently it prevents certain cardiovascular disorders. Highly recommended for hypertension, arteriosclerosis, and vascular diseases.

• **Corn.** It has the most important fat content among all grains. Its active elements act directly on the thyroid gland to slow it down. However, its lack of vitamin B3 (PP) makes it a good complementary food.

• **Millet.** With a significant percentage of phosphorus, iron, and vitamin A, it is highly recommended against mental fatigue, nervous depression, asthenia and anemia.

• **Wheat.** It is the most commonly grown grain in the southern regions of Europe. It is richer in minerals (sulfur, calcium, phosphorus, iron, magnesium, potassium, silicon, sodium, etc.) and also has a large number of trace elements and vitamins (B1, B2, B12, D, E, K, and PP). It is used to make all types of pasta and somewhat exotic dishes such as bulgur, couscous, and seitan.

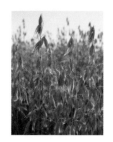

Grains, for their many properties, must be part of any balanced diet.

Buckwheat

Despite its name, this is not a wheat itself. Its use, however, is highly recommended, as it has more calcium than wheat and several essential amino acids such as tryptophan, which is present in animal proteins.

Raw or cooked?

We should always try to eat grains and starches raw, since when they are heated they lose some of their vitamins and minerals. But if cooking is necessary (as for rice) try blanching or steaming. Use the water you cook them in as bases for soups or broths.

VEGETABLES

Raw or cooked, they consist of ninety percent water (and salts). Vegetables alone represent a small but powerful energy value. They are the primary source of vitamins (A and C, especially), minerals (sodium, calcium, magnesium, etc.) and fiber.

Furthermore, their alkaline makeup neutralizes acidification caused by foods rich in proteins and they facilitate the removal of waste accumulation that in the long run often causes poisoning.

During childhood and adolescence, protein intake is important and often believed to be a complementary food, but this is not the case so it is important to accustom the palate to a variety of flavors, against fast food and its exaggerated effects. Vegetables are interesting at any age, and in old age, they become the center of the diet because there are less caloric needs and an increase in constipation and digestive disorders.

FRUIT

They are one of the best sources of carbohydrates (mostly fructose, glucose, and levulose), water (80 to 90%), minerals, vitamins (especially C, common in kiwi, guava, blackcurrant, lemon, orange, mango, and strawberry), fiber (cellulose) and acids that aid digestion and protect vitamins.

MILK AND DAIRY PRODUCTS

Lately there is a tendency to question the importance of milk (especially cow's milk) as a staple food for adults. It is true that it provides calcium (which can also be obtained from fish, cauliflower, turnips, seaweed—in higher amounts—nuts, lettuce, and leafy greens, etc.), but the absorption of cow's milk is far from wholesome.

Tips for eating fruit

• Fruit must always be **in season**. Distrust oranges in summer or plums in December: either they have been imported from distant countries or they have been kept in refrigerated containers. In both cases, the fruit has been damaged and lost most of its nutritional properties.

• Fruit should be eaten **ripe** and chewed carefully to avoid poor digestion that could cause gas.

• Due to the use of pesticides, preservatives, and brighteners, fruit should be **washed** thoroughly with water and lemon juice before eating. If you are unsure, it is better to peel it.

• Do not eat fruits with bites, bruises or cuts, however small, it is very likely that they contain **insecticides**.

• It is better to eat fruit **before meals** for better digestion. If you want, once a week do a cleansing diet by eating only fruits.

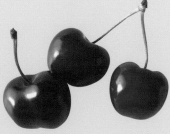

Moreover, the enzyme capable of metabolizing milk gradually disappears after age three. Milk ensures a more than satisfactory supply of vitamins (A, B12, D, and E), proteins, and minerals, but it also contains a considerable proportion of fatty acids that are not good for those with high cholesterol, liver problems, or gallbladder disorders.

Yogurt and kefir are produced by bacterial fermentation of milk, very similar to what gastric juices do in our stomach. They should be eaten regularly: to help food absorption and regulate gastric juices and intestinal flora.

Butter, obtained from cream that condenses on the surface of milk, has 84% fat, 15% water, and 0.5% carbohydrates as well as vitamins A and D.

Given that it contains preservatives, and it is an unhealthy fat, **margarine** is not a good substitute for butter. Use **buttercream** instead (62% water, 31% fat, 4% carbohydrates, and 3% proteins). Like butter, it contains vitamins A and D. However, these three dairy products are not suitable for people with a sensitive stomach or liver, or who suffer from high cholesterol.

Cheeses are usually classified as follows: *fresh* cheeses that have 70–80% moisture, 10% fat and vitamin C (cottage cheese, Burgos, Villalón, Mató, etc.) They are recommended for obese persons or those who suffer from arteriosclerosis or high cholesterol. *Soft*, with 50–60% moisture, and richer in protein and fat. *Cured* cheeses that have 35–40% moisture and 30% protein are not recommended for people with kidney failure, digestive disorders, and obesity. And finally, *veined* cheeses that have 40–45% moisture, B vitamins, and a considerable fat content.

EGGS

Eggs are a beneficial food; the yolk is rich in proteins, lipids, nitrogen, and phosphorus, vitamins A and D, iron, and lecithin. The white, meanwhile, is for the most part protein. They are preferable to meat, but people suffering from the same disorders as in the case of milk should avoid eating eggs.

LEGUMES

Legumes contain vitamins, carbohydrates, minerals (calcium, iron, and magnesium) and 17 to 25% protein. It is a similar or even higher percentage than meat and fish (as in the case of soybeans, 36%). Their essential amino acids (especially lysine) are supplemented by grains (sulfur-containing amino acids), so eating grains and legumes together allows you to better use their proteins.

Tips for eating vegetables

• Legumes have a lot of non-digestible substances (saponines, alkaloids, etc.).
• To avoid indigestion and flatulence, soak them for several hours before cooking. They must simmer for a long time so that they are completely cooked.
• To reinforce their protein power, pair them with vegetables and serve with any type of grain.
• When eating, chew them well and salivate.

OILS AND NUTS

Vegetable oils are one of the most important sources of energy in our body. They are mostly made up of monounsaturated fat, which does not affect cholesterol levels. They are used as dressing or for cooking. Using olive oil in Mediterranean countries is directly related to much lower rates of heart disease than in countries where animal fats are often used for cooking.

Nuts can be used to substitute for meat protein when eaten frequently in certain amounts. Their fat and protein content is much higher than other vegetables (except soybeans). Furthermore, they are better than meat because they do not create waste during metabolism (urea, uric acid, etc.), nor undergo a decomposition process before we ingest them, and we can eat them raw without worrying about parasites and bacteria.

Daily dietary needs

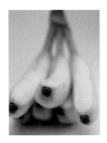

Most food provides the energy needed to perform all vital functions.

These are the three nutrient classification categories that the World Health Organization (WHO) established:

• **Body building nutrients,** responsible for the production, maintenance and repair of tissues. Proteins and minerals belong in this group.

• **Energy nutrients** that supply the energy needed for the body to perform all its functions. This category consists of carbohydrates, fats, and, with some exceptions, also proteins.

• **Protective nutrients** that regulate metabolism. This group consists of vitamins, minerals, and water.

As shown, the largest category is made up of energy nutrients. Most foods, when ingested and broken down into nutrients, provide enough energy to perform our body's maintenance and regeneration needs. This energy, from a nutritional point, is measured in calories.

PROTEINS

Proteins enable the production of new cells and tissue regeneration. Nutritionally, their importance depends on the rate at which they can be utilized by the body. Their absorption will be higher or lower depending on the type of amino acids that constitute them. The human body is able to synthesize a good portion of proteins. The rest, known as "essential amino acids," must be obtained from food.

What is a serving?

When determining how much of each type of food should be eaten daily, dietitians speak of "serving size," which is calculated from the eating habits of different social groups and survey data on nutrition. Their validity is very relative because each person must follow the kind of diet that best suits their individual physical needs (weight, muscle mass, body type . . .), and mental needs (relationship with food). However, serving sizes can help us organize our weekly menus.

Examples of a serving size

· Starches
  1 slice (60 g) bread
  ½ cup (75 g) of rice, noodles
    or macaroni, raw
  ½ cup (150 g) potatoes

· Fats
  10 ml of oil (one tablespoon)
  8 (25 g) walnuts

· Fruit
  1 cup (200 g) pears, apples, peaches, etc.
  4 tangerines

4 apricots
½ cup (100 g) strawberries
  or cherries

· Milk
  1 slice of melon
  1 cup (250ml) milk
  2 yogurts
  2 slices (50 g) of cheese

· Vegetables
  1 cup (200 g) salad
  1 cup (200 g) fresh vegetables
  2 carrots
  2 tomatoes

Milk, cheese, eggs, fish, and meat provide all necessary proteins.

The most important are lysine, methionine, and tryptophan, which are also the most difficult to obtain. Therefore, include various foods that provide the necessary proteins when eaten together.

CARBOHYDRATES

They are our most important sources of energy. They are abundant in fruit, milk, grains, vegetables, legumes, and honey. They are divided into three groups: monosaccharides (fructose, glucose, and galactose, easy to digest), disaccharides (sucrose, maltose, and lactose, harder to digest) and polysaccharides (starch, cellulose, or fiber, much harder to digest).

Refined carbohydrates, which are commonly found in baked goods, provide hardly any nutrients and their caloric value is huge. Eating them is related with tooth decay, diabetes, and hypertension. A very high-fiber, vegetarian diet ensures good elimination of toxins.

Protein-rich foods

Almonds	16.9 g/100 g
Peanuts	24.3 g/100 g
Yeast extract	39.7 g/100 g
Wheat germ	26.5 g/100 g
Oatmeal	12.4 g/100 g
Wholemeal	13.2 g/100 g
Soybean meal	36.8 g/100 g
Eggs	12.3 g/100 g
Cooked lentils	7.6 g/100 g
Brazil nuts	12 g/100 g
Pistachios	19.3 g/100 g
Cheese ball	26 g/100 g
Manchego cheese	35.1 g/100 g
Cottage cheese	13.6 g/100 g

Recommended Daily Allowance: 65-75 g (men) and 58-63 g (women)

Fiber-rich foods

Almonds	14.3 g/100 g
Peanuts	8.1 g/100 g
Prunes	16.1 g/100 g
Coconut flakes	23.5 g/100 g
Dates	8.7 g/100 g
Raspberries	7.4 g/100 g
Wholemeal flour	7 g/100 g
Soybean flour	11.9 g/100 g
Whole wheat flour	9.6 g/100 g
Dried figs	18.5 g/100 g
Green beans	7.4 g/100 g
Brazil nuts	9 g/100 g
Dried apricots	24 g/100 g
Dried peaches	14.3 g/100 g
Whole wheat bread	8.5 g/100 g
Parsley	9.1 g/100 g
Bran	44 g/100 g

FATS

Despite their bad press, eating them moderately is essential for maintaining the body in perfect conditions because they provide energy and heat, they are stored in fat cells as reserve fuel, they protect some organs, and guarantee the absorption of fat soluble vitamins (A, D, K, and E).

There are two types of fats: saturated and unsaturated. *Saturated* fats have a solid consistency at room temperature, they are mostly found in animal products (cream, cheese, butter, eggs), and they contain *harmful* cholesterol, which, in excess, can increase the risk of coronary heart disease. Unsaturated fats consist of two groups: monounsaturated, found in vegetable oils and do not affect cholesterol levels, and polyunsaturated, which tend to reduce cholesterol levels.

VITAMINS

Our body cannot synthesize all the necessary vitamins to regulate metabolism, grow, and regenerate damaged tissues. Therefore, we have to turn to certain foods that contain vitamins.

• **Vitamin A.** Also called "retinol," is responsible for skin regeneration, mucous membranes, and eyes. It is found only in animal products, though the body can produce it from "carotene" or pro-vitamin A found in many green or orange vegetables (such as the popular carrots). If not taken in sufficient amounts, we can experience fatigue, sore eyes, and night blindness.

Fatty acid content (per 100 g)

Vegetable oils	Saturated	Monounsaturated	Polyunsaturated	Nuts	Saturated
Peanut	19.7	50.1	29.8	Almonds	8.3
Safflower	10.7	13.2	75.5	Hazelnuts	7.5
Sunflower	13.7	33.3	52.3	Peanuts	15.2
Corn	17.2	30.7	51.6	Chestnuts	18.2
Olive	14.7	73	11.7	Coconut	83
Soy	14.7	25.4	59.4	Walnuts	11.4
				Brazil nuts	26.7

• **B vitamins** help transform nutrients into energy and ensure red blood cell formation. They must be in a balanced ratio, because if there is an excess of one, the others may be deficient. Let's look:

a. Folic acid. It is found in leafy greens so eat a plate of salad per day. Its deficiency is very common among pregnant women or among women taking oral contraceptives, there may be tiredness, anemia, and depression.

b. Vitamin B1 or thiamine. Needed for breaking down carbohydrates.

c. Vitamin B2 or riboflavin. Especially present in milk, it breaks down when exposed to sunlight. Its deficiency can result in dry lips and eye redness. Raw almonds are good for riboflavin.

Foods rich in vitamin A

Sorrel	2,150 mg/100 g
Watercress	500 mg/100 g
Baked sweet potato	667 mg/100 g
Cooked broccoli	417 mg/100 g
Green dandelion leaves	2,333 mg/100 g
Endive	334 mcg/100 g
Cooked spinach	1000 mg/100 g
Eggs	140 mg/100 g
Milk	40 mg/100 g
Mango	200 mg/100 g
Butter	985 mg/100 g
Melon	334 mg/100 g
Dried apricots	600 mg/100 g
Parsley	1,166 mg/100 g
Edam cheese	410 mg/100 g
Carrot	2,000 mg/100 g

Recommended Daily Allowance: 750 mg

Foods rich in vitamin B_1

Almonds	0.67 mg/100 g
Hazelnuts	0.40 mg/100 g
Peanuts	0.90 mg/100 g
Oats	0.55 mg/100 g
Yeast extract	3.10 mg/100 g
Wheat germ	1.45 mg/100 g
Raw peas	0.30 mg/100 g
Oatmeal	0.50 mg/100 g
Wholemeal	0.46 mg/100 g
Soybean meal	0.80 mg/100 g
Dried kidney beans	0.60 mg/100 g
Walnuts	0.30 mg/100 g
Brazil nuts	1 mg/100 g
Whole wheat bread	0.26 mg/100 g
Bran	0.89 mg/100 g
Dry soybean	1.10 mg/100 g

Recommended daily amount: 0.9 to 1.2 mg

Monounsaturated	Polyunsaturated
71.6	19.6
81.1	10.9
50.1	29.8
39.2	41.9
7	1.8
16.3	71.4
34.3	39

A balanced diet

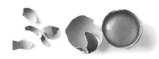

Foods rich in vitamin B2

Almonds	0.92 mg/100 g
Cooked broccoli	0.20 mg/100 g
Brie and similar cheeses	0.60 mg/100 g
Mushrooms	0.40 mg/100 g
Raw spinach	0.29 mg/100 g
Wheat germ	0.81 mg/100 g
Eggs	0.47 mg/100 g
Milk	0.20 mg/100 g
Manchego cheese	0.50 mg/100 g
Yogurt	0.26 mg/100 g

Recommended daily amount: 1.5 to 1.7 mg

Foods rich in vitamin B3

Almonds	6.5 mg/100 g
Roasted peanuts	16 mg/100 g
Mushrooms	4 mg/100 g
Dates	2 mg/100 g
Wheat germ	5.8 mg/100 g
Baked beans	3 mg/100 g
Wholemeal flour	5.6 mg/100 g
Popcorn	2.2 mg/100 g

Recommended daily amount: 15 to 18 mg

Foods rich in vitamin B6

Avocado	0.42 mg/100 g
Hazelnuts	0.55 mg/100 g
Peanuts	1 mg/100 g
Soybean meal	0.57 mg/100 g
Egg	0.3 mg/100 g
Yeast	4.20 mg/100 g
Brewer's yeast	1.20 mg/100 g
Bananas	0.51 mg/100 g
Raw carrot	0.20 mg/100 g

Recommended Daily Allowance: 2 mg

d. Vitamin B_3, niacin, or nicotinic acid. Our bodies can synthesize it with the help of tryptophan, an essential amino acid found mainly in milk, eggs, . . . and the humble peanut. Its deficiency causes irritability, nervousness, and pellagra.

e. Vitamin B_6 or pyridoxine. It is essential for pregnant women, women who take oral contraceptives, or those suffering premenstrual symptoms. If taken with vitamin B2 and magnesium its effectiveness increases. It is highly perishable because it is destroyed by heat and food preparation. If not taken in sufficient quantities, there can be symptoms of anemia, fatigue, depression, migraines, and nervous disorders.

f. Vitamin B_{12}. It is found in some seaweed, but it is mostly found in animal-based foods. If a strict vegetarian diet without eggs or dairy products is followed, this vitamin should be taken as supplements. Sun baths in the earlier part of the day are good for its absorption. Its deficiency can cause paralysis and anemia.

• Vitamin C or ascorbic acid. It maintains connective tissue in good condition and allows iron absorption. Prevents many diseases and is helpful in postoperative recovery. This vitamin is highly recommended during stressful situations or if you are battling tobacco, alcohol, or coffee addiction. It breaks down very easily, especially when exposed to air or heat. Its deficiency causes a weakening of connective tissue, bleeding, poor wound healing, and weakened immune system. To avoid these issues, eat a lot of fruits and vegetables.

• **Vitamin D.** Essential for the absorption of calcium and phosphorus, it is generated by the effect of sunlight on the skin. It is also found in dairy products, eggs, and margarine, although in smaller quantities. Its deficiency can eventually lead to rickets and bone degeneration.

• **Vitamin E.** It forms and maintains body cells and wound healing. It is found in cold pressed vegetable oils (and their derivatives), grains, eggs, and nuts. Contributes to longevity. Its deficiency can cause fatigue and anemia.

• **Vitamin K.** helps blood clotting. It is found in vegetables, grains, and seaweed. Its deficiency is rare.

MINERALS

These nutrients cannot be synthesized by the human body. They are needed in varying amounts: while our intake of calcium, iron, potassium, and magnesium should be high, our intake of zinc and iodine needs to be much lower. They cannot be absorbed in their purest form, but in the form of organic salts made from plant and animal organisms.

• **Calcium.** 99% of the calcium in the human body (which is no more than 1.5% of total weight) is in the bones and teeth. Calcium contributes to blood clotting, heart muscle contraction, and nerve function, allowing transmission of nerve impulses.

Foods rich in vitamin B$_{12}$

Seaweed	trace amounts
Brie and similar cheese	1.2 mg/100g
Yeast extract	0.5 mg/100 g
Eggs	1.7 mg/100 g
Milk	0.3 mg/100 g
Butter	trace amounts
Cream	0.2 mg/100 g
Cheese ball	1.5 mg/100 g
Manchego cheese	1.5 mg/100 g
Cottage cheese	0.5 mg/100 g
Yolk	4.9 mg/100 g
Yogurt	trace amounts

Recommended daily amount: from 1 to 2 mg

Foods rich in vitamin C

Cooked broccoli	34 mg/100 g
Raw cabbage	60 mg/100 g
Raspberries	25 mg/100 g
Blackcurrant	200 mg/100 g
Kiwi	500 mg/100 g
Lichis	40 mg/100 g
Lemon	80 mg/100 g
Mangos	30 mg/100 g
Oranges	50 mg/100 g
Parsley	150 mg/100 g
Red peppers	204 mg/100 g
Green peppers	100 mg/100 g
Grapefruit	40 mg/100 g
Radishes	25 mg/100 g

Recommended daily amount: 30 mg

Caloric intake

1 g protein	4 calories
1 g carbohydrate	4 calories
1 g of fat	9 calories

Foods rich in vitamin E

Virgin olive oil	8.0 mg/100 g
Peanuts	15 mg/100 g
Raw cauliflower	2 mg/100 g
Raw spinach	6 mg/100 g
Wheat germ	30 mg/100 g
Raw peas	2.1 mg/100 g
Whole wheat flour	2.2 mg/100 g
Tender green beans	3.6 mg/100 g

Recommended daily amount: 12 mg

Foods rich in zinc

Almonds	3.1 mg/100 g
Hazelnuts	2.4 mg/100 g
Peanuts	3 mg/100 g
Wholemeal flour	3 mg/100 g
Walnuts	3 mg/100 g
Brie	3 mg/100 g
Manchego cheese	4 mg/100 g

Recommended daily amount: 15 mg

Foods rich in magnesium

Almonds	260 mg/100 g
Peanuts	180 mg/100 g
Wheat germ	300 mg/100 g
Oatmeal	110 mg/100 g
Wholemeal flour	140 mg/100 g
Soybean meal	240 mg/100 g
Cooked dried beans	65 mg/100 g
Millet	162 mg/100 g
Walnuts	130 mg/100 g
Brazil nuts	410 mg/100 g
Dried apricots	65 mg/100 g
Whole wheat bread	93 mg/100 g
Bran	520 mg/100 g

Recommended Daily Allowance: 340 mg

Its absorption depends on vitamin D. Its deficiency causes neurasthenia, insomnia, irritability, and leg cramps. It is important to ensure their absorption during childhood and adolescence, otherwise growth problems and rickets may occur.

• **Zinc.** Although present in many foods, the body does not absorb it in large quantities. Its presence is minimal but it increases libido, it is found in semen, and it is the most commonly found mineral in the prostate.

• **Phosphorus.** Along with calcium, it forms the mineral substrate in bones and teeth. In excess it is quite dangerous, so it must be supplemented with calcium and zinc.

• **Iron.** Ensures oxygen flow in the blood, and forms hemoglobin. It is found in our enzymes. It transforms carotene into vitamin A. Vitamin C facilitates its absorption. If not taken in sufficient amounts, there is fatigue and anemia. As a supplement, it can destroy a significant percentage of vitamin E.

• **Magnesium.** It allows cells to retain potassium and regulates the functioning of vitamin B6. It is the catalyst for many biological functions (nutrient absorption, energy release, transmission of nerve impulses, synthesis of body compounds, muscular contraction). In excess, it is noticeably laxative.

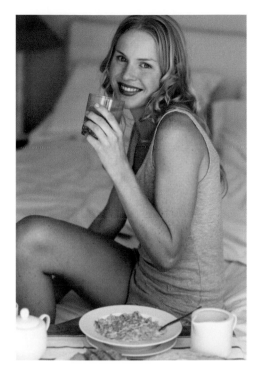

Foods rich in folic acid

Almonds	96 mg/100 g
Baked sweet potato	140 mg/100 g
Raw cabbage	90 mg/100 g
Cooked Brussels sprouts	100 mg/100 g
Endive	330 mg/100 g
Wheat germ	330 mg/100 g
Yeast	1,250 mg/100 g
Bran	260 mg/100 g

Recommended Daily Allowance: 200 mg

Foods rich in potassium

Almonds	860 mg/100 g
Yeast extract	2600 mg/100 g
Dried beans	1,500 mg/100 g
Soybean meal	1,660 mg/100 g
Dried figs	1,010 mg/100 g
Dried peaches	1,100 mg/100 g
Dried apricots	1,880 mg/100 g
French fries	1,000 mg/100 g
Parsley	1.880 mg/100 g
Dry soybean	1,900 mg/100 g

Daily Value: 3,000 mg

Iron-rich foods

Almonds	4.4 mg/100 g
Bitter chocolate	6.8 mg/100 g
Wheat germ	10 mg/100 g
Soy flour	6.9 mg/100 g
Dried figs	4.2 mg/100 g
Dried beans	7.3 mg/100 g
Millet	6.8 mg/100 g
Dried peaches	6.8 mg/100 g
Bran	12.9 mg/100 g
Egg yolk	6.1 mg/100 g

Recommended daily amount: 10 to 12 mg

Its deficiency causes muscle cramps, spasms, insomnia and depression.

• **Sodium and potassium.** Regulate body fluids and water retention. Sodium deficiency is very unlikely, since food supplies it in sufficient quantities. Eating salty foods can prevent the absorption of potassium and increase the risk for hypertension.

• **Iodine.** Regulates the thyroid gland. It is found in seaweed or crops grown on iodinated soil. Although its presence in the human body is very small, its deficiency can cause thyroid disease, high cholesterol level in the blood, and affect physical and mental development.

Top ten foods for a well-balanced diet

In this section you will find charts for a balanced diet. It is not intended as a restricted diet because, as you will remember, sudden changes in eating habits tend not to last very long.

What we suggest is a series of small changes to eat smart without starving yourself or giving up the pleasures of food.

Because we eat several times a day, every day of our lives, it is important to know the properties of each food, its therapeutic properties, and its relationship to other natural products.

In his book *La alimentación equilibrada* (Ed. Océano, 2002) Dr. Barnet Meltzer cautions: "The most affordable disease is the one that never happens. You have to learn to take care of yourself in order to catch it before it catches up with you." Poor eating habits not only promote physical illnesses, they can also contribute to depression, anxiety, and decreased libido.

These charts have been designed for everyone to take control of their eating by focusing on their specific needs.

Each person has a predisposition to specific illnesses, with strengths and weaknesses. Therefore it is very important for you to know your own body. The best personal doctor you can count on is yourself!

Health begins at the table, and by bringing natural and wholesome products to the table, we can live longer and better. It is up to us whether our foods are our allies or enemies. Let's explore a bit more:

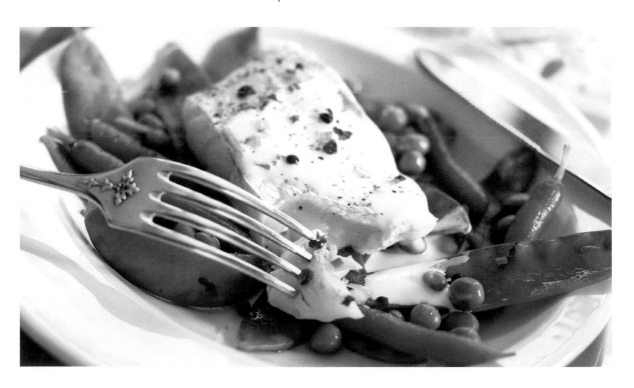

Living without heartburn: acidic and alkaline foods

Combining meat, fish, milk, eggs, etc., gives us not only proteins but also acidic toxins that attack our bodies. An excess of acidic foods increases oxidation (aging) of the cells and promotes the formation of cholesterol in the arteries. A vegetarian diet, however, leads to an alkaline biochemistry for health and wellness.

"Heartburn" is a disorder that many of us chose to ignore.

Excessive acidity increases the risk of cancer, arteriosclerosis, and even Parkinson's disease.

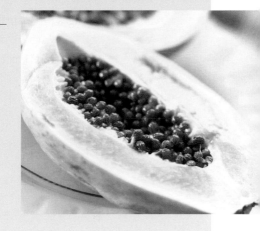

Highly alkaline foods	Highly acidic foods
1. Almonds	1. Offal
2. Broccoli	2. Pork
3. Sprouts	3. Eggs
4. Sunflower	4. Seafood
5. Papaya	5. Smoked fish
6. Potatoes	6. Oily fish
7. Watermelon	7. Chicken
8. Soy (tofu)	8. Veal
9. Leafy greens	
10. Carrots	

* More information in the book: *Vivir sin acidez*, ed. Océano Ámbar.

Energy-rich foods and energy-deficient foods

When choosing foods it is important not to focus on their caloric value, but rather on their nutritional content. This list includes natural products with the highest levels of phytonutrients, a treasure trove of antioxidants that slow the aging process and help prevent inflammatory and carcinogenic disease.

On the other hand, there are energy-deficient foods. Oftentimes, chronic fatigue is due more to what we eat than to our daily activity. Fatigue, in this sense, is an alarm that warns us that something is not working properly in our body. Let's see what falls where in nutritional categories.

The top 10 energy-rich foods	The top 10 energy-deficient foods
1. Spirulina	1. Alcohol
2. Fruit smoothies	2. Chocolates and sweets
3. Broccoli and other crucifers	3. Canned fruit
4. Citrus	4. Eggs
5. Veggie burgers	5. Lobster and other seafood
6. Royal jelly	6. White bread and butter
7. Whole wheat bread	7. Potato chips and pretzels
8. Roasted potatoes	8. Fried chicken
9. Reishi and shiitake mushrooms	9. Dairy products
10. Tempeh	10. Beef and pork products

Aphrodisiacs

In every culture, food has been associated to libido and sexual stamina. Modern medicine proves that indeed there are certain local products that stimulate our sex drive. We know, for instance, that vitamin E, magnesium, potassium, and zinc help regulate sex hormones, and vitamin B$_3$ or niacin increases blood flow and promotes erection in men. Later on we will explore the most virtuous foods; this list is just a preview:

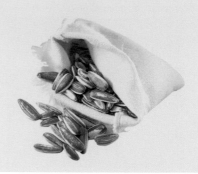

The top 10 most aphrodisiac foods

1. Avocado
2. Almonds
3. Celery
4. Onions and tomatoes
5. Chilies, spices, and herbs
6. Asparagus and artichokes
7. Fruit and nuts
8. Romaine lettuce
9. Whole wheat bread
10. Pumpkin and sunflower seeds

Serotonin enhancers

Serotonin is an important neurotransmitter with ability to lift up our mood. Therefore, not having this substance causes depressive disorders and irritability. Many antidepressant drugs artificially increase serotonin levels with significant side effects.

Once again, foods that come from Mother Nature are the best medicine. It is known that tryptophan increases brain serotonin, so eating foods rich in this amino acid elevates serotonin levels, while increasing endorphins and other neurotransmitters.

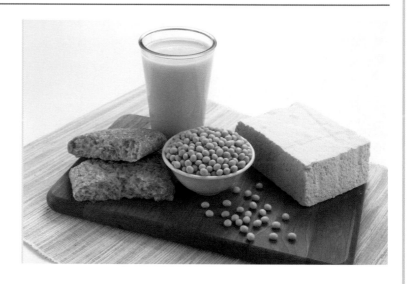

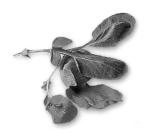

Top 10 foods rich in tryptophan

1. Celery
2. Watercress
3. Broccoli
4. Alfalfa sprouts
5. Cauliflower
6. Chicory
7. Spinach
8. Soy products
9. Beet
10. Carrot

Foods rich in phenylalanine and tyrosine

Phenylalanine and tyrosine are two important amino acids that help influence (and determine) our mood. People who suffer from depression often have low levels of both. Phenylalanine is an essential component in the production of norepinephrine, a hormone that is often depleted by stress in the adrenal glands. Tyrosine regulates an important balance between the thyroid, pituitary, and adrenal glands.

Let's see what foods contribute to our positive feelings.

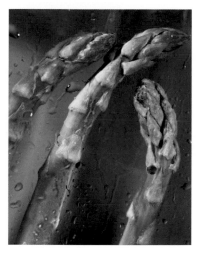

Top 10 foods rich in phenylalanine

1. Avocados
2. Almonds
3. Spinach
4. Legumes
5. Peanut butter
6. Parsley
7. Pineapple
8. Soy products
9. Miso soup
10. Tomatoes

Top 10 foods rich in tyrosine

1. Avocados
2. Almonds and almond butter
3. Asparagus
4. Spinach
5. Romaine lettuce
6. Peanut butter
7. Apples
8. Soy products
9. Watermelon
10. Carrots

Folic acid

Folic acid plays a crucial role in brain chemistry and in nourishing the blood and strengthening the immune system. For those of us who like to enjoy life, folic acid increases levels of S-adenosylmethionine, which in turn increases serotonin and dopamine levels.

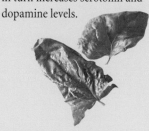

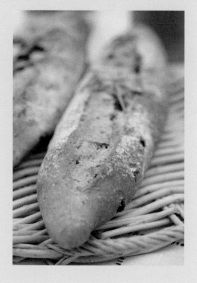

Top 10 foods rich in folic acid

1. Broccoli
2. Grains and whole wheat bread
3. Kale and beet
4. Asparagus
5. Spinach
6. Wheat germ
7. Legumes
8. Lentils and beans
9. Brewer's yeast
10. Soy products

A balanced diet

Vitamin B$_6$

A deficiency in this vitamin negatively affects serotonin in the body. There is a particular deficiency of this vitamin in women with PMS or menopause. Further on in this book, we will look closely at the most important sources of vitamin B$_6$.

Top 10 foods rich in vitamin B$_6$

1. Avocados
2. Brown rice
3. Spinach
4. Legumes
5. Lentils
6. Brewer's yeast
7. Walnuts
8. Sunflower seeds
9. Bananas
10. Tofu and other soy products

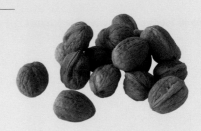

Magnesium and zinc

Magnesium is one of the most therapeutic components that nature can give us. In addition to mitigating irritability, nervousness, and muscle tension, it is very beneficial for treating disorders associated with fibromyalgia. Zinc helps calm the nerves and prevents anxiety disorders. These are two minerals that are essential to the health of body and mind.

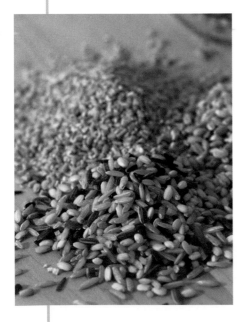

Foods rich in magnesium

1. Avocados
2. Almonds
3. Brown rice
4. Citrus
5. Lentils
6. Potatoes
7. Sesame seeds
8. Tofu and soy products
9. Leafy greens
10. Carrots

Foods rich in zinc

1. Almonds
2. Oatmeal
3. Peanuts
4. Whole grains
5. Peas
6. Dry peas
7. Lima beans
8. Brazil nuts
9. Pecans
10. Pumpkin seeds

Pyridoxine

Also called vitamin B_6, pyridoxine protects neurotransmitters by metabolizing glutamic acid, which transmits information from any part of the body to the brain. Besides this function, vitamin B_6 deficiency is often associated with different diseases such as asthma, cardiovascular disorders, kidney stones, and epileptic seizures.

Top 10 foods rich in pyridoxine (vitamin B_6)

1. Avocados
2. Brown rice
3. Chickpeas
4. Pinto beans
5. Lentils
6. Brewer's yeast
7. Walnuts
8. Sunflower seeds
9. Bananas
10. Tofu and other soy products

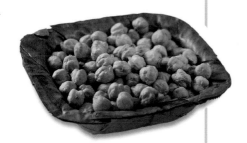

Thiamine

Also called vitamin B_1, thiamine helps regulate carbohydrate metabolism, energy production, and nerve cell function. Moreover, thiamine optimizes acetylcholine, the neurotransmitter that prevents memory loss.

Alcohol disables thiamine, so avoid drinking as much as possible and choose products rich in vitamin B_1.

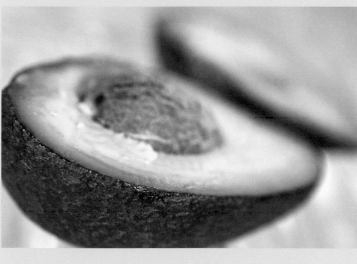

Top 10 foods rich in vitamin B_1

1. Avocados
2. Brown rice
3. Spinach
4. Legumes
5. Lentils
6. Brewer's yeast
7. Walnuts
8. Sunflower seeds
9. Bananas
10. Tofu and other soy products

Superfoods to improve your sex life

Throughout the book, you will see aphrodisiac foods show up sporadically. We devote a chapter to them because of their connection to superfoods and general interest in this topic. Remember that there are multiple factors (age, muscle mass and weight, metabolic rhythm, diet, lifestyle, etc.) that make aphrodisiacs work for some people, but not for others. Experts agree that aphrodisiac foods or products are quite a superstition throughout the ages, but it is harder to get them to agree on what food to eat in order to enjoy better sex, especially after the emergence of a lot of new energy supplements. We have summarized typical aphrodisiac foods along with the latest findings in two major sections:

1) Restorative foods that are essential for energy and nutritional balance.
2) "Sexy" foods, with more immediate effects and variable results.

REGULAR MEALS

The balance in our sex hormones is closely related to how we metabolize all other hormones (which control cell growth and regeneration, in addition to the immune, digestive, and respiratory systems). So to enjoy optimum health benefits, we need to include all the nutrients, some of which are more related to sexual health.

Let's take a look at these nutrients and the richest sources of them. Remember also that when we skip a meal or eat too much, all we end up with is fatigue.

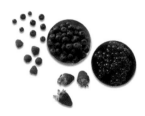

Some foods provide us with certain nutrients related to sexual health.

A key to enhancing stamina is having the right blood sugar level. To do so:

• Combine protein, carbohydrates, and fiber in each meal. Eat less in quantity, but more frequently, about 4 to 5 times a day.
• Reduce stimulants (tea, coffee, soft drinks).
• Eat more fresh foods.

STRESS, DEPRESSION, FATIGUE

To mitigate the effects of stress, bring in some basic lifestyle changes to prevent anxiety and nervousness, including:

• Deep breathing and adequate rest.
• Eliminate or reduce your intake of alcohol, coffee, or other drugs.
• Making sure to include three essential nutrients in your diet: **vitamin C** (citrus, peppers, blueberries or red berries, kiwi, watermelon); **vitamin B$_3$** (vegetables and leafy greens, rice, peanuts, wheat germ) and **magnesium** (whole grains, nuts, vegetables, and leafy greens, all fruits).

Mild depression, mood changes, or seasonal affective disorders strongly affect sexual appetite and erotic behavior (erectile disorders, loss of libido, or inability to reach an orgasm).

Giving in to the occasional sweet such as ice cream, for example, is very uplifting: a "guilty pleasure" that enhances our serotonin levels. But through dopamine, it can reduce testosterone levels. Dopamine acts as a neurotransmitter and requires protein to synthesize. Hence our need for a rich and varied diet.

Vitamin B_6, which is related to the synthesis of serotonin, is necessary to lift the spirits. Vitamins B_9 and B_{12} are also needed to synthesize dopamine. Zinc, magnesium, and selenium also help.

SEX AND RELAXATION: THE THYROID GLAND

Under stressful conditions, blood thickens and causes headaches (which have become the most common excuse for avoiding sexual intercourse). Daily worry affects desire and sexual appetite, so you have to put worry aside as much as possible before going to bed. Rest and sleep play an important role in our libido.

Sex is also a great stress reliever, so try to engage in games and sexual activities with your partner if you suffer from stress or insomnia. Sleep quality improves with sexual practice.

The thyroid regulates metabolism and energy. If it does not function properly, then libido also lowers. Have your doctor check that it is functioning correctly, especially if you experience weight gain and a lower sex drive.

Foods rich in iodine (necessary for the thyroid to produce tyrosine) are kombu seaweed and blue-green algae, shellfish and seafood, cabbage, radishes and its leaf, fruit juice, melon, cucumber, and spinach.

Iodine-rich foods promote good thyroid function and therefore a healthy sex drive.

Testosterone

Testosterone plays an important role in our libido and it is even present in women. Leydig cells in the testes of healthy men produce about 7 mg of testosterone per day. But stress affects them directly as precursor hormones (cortisol and testosterone) originate from the same place. Imagine a car reaching a crossroad and it must choose between turning left to manage stress or turn right to produce testosterone. If there is any stressor that needs to be controlled, the car always turn first to the left.

Testosterone is essential for sperm production, fertility, erection,

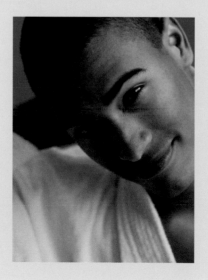

and to maintain and regulate sex drive. The less testosterone there is, the more fatigue there is, which is typical among middle-aged men and young professionals. A decrease in testosterone usually affects men (andropause) just as women are affected by menopause. It has been found that this decrease causes men to suffer from both psychological and physical changes in their late forties or mid-fifties, such as lacking goals or concentration at work and a lack of interest in family and close friends, and low self-esteem.

LOSS OF LIBIDO IN MEN

Sex hormones are closely related to hormones released by endocrine glands. For example, adrenaline from the adrenal glands controls stress, while tyrosine from the thyroid gland regulates metabolism and energy production.

If the balance is altered in any of these glands that are essential for proper body functioning, then it would directly harm the rest; for example, the ovaries and testes. So fatigue, anxiety, and emotional pressures become the main cause of loss of libido and of typical comments such as: "I am very tired" or "Not tonight, dear."

PROSTATE

Today, prostate health is associated with erectile dysfunction. Inflammation of the prostate has become so common that most doctors assume it is directly related to the male aging process, but if good nutritional guidelines are followed, this should not be a problem. The prostate gland, which is the size of a walnut, opens into the urethra (from the bladder) and secretes a fluid that makes up semen. Excessive enlargement of the prostate (benign prostatic hyperplasia or BPH) is quite common in men ages twenty to sixty. If the size of the prostate increases then the bladder neck gets completely clogged, causing some difficulty urinating. BPH can affect men's ability to achieve an erection.

Dietary estrogens (isoflavonoids, flavonoids, and lignin) can help reduce the incidence of BPH. BPH affects the Japanese population much less, since their intake of soy (tofu, tempeh, miso, or soy beverages) is very high.

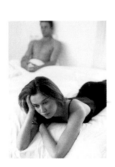

Fatigue, anxiety, and emotional pressures are the main cause of loss of libido.

Zinc is also recommended in foods, but in case of BPH about 50 mg per day can be taken in supplement form. Do not exceed 80 mg zinc from all sources ingested.

LOSS OF LIBIDO IN WOMEN

As we can see, both men and women need hormonal balance to ensure regular and satisfying sexual lives. Any hormonal imbalance affects our sexual activity, which is why you should know which hormones are related to libido. Women also produce testosterone, and not only from the ovaries, because the adrenal glands, brain, skin, and fat reserves are also responsible for it. So it is women who suffer most from the effects of menopause, as they have less testosterone fat reserves. To balance testosterone levels, eat foods rich in zinc and vitamin B_6.

Estrogen and progesterone imbalances contribute to loss of libido by interrupting, shortening, or lengthening the menstrual cycle. Those who suffer a strong premenstrual syndrome (PMS) are more likely to lack sexual appetite, because there are physical and mental changes that result in mood swings and loss of self-esteem.

Erection troubles: Viagra and natural alternatives

There is a strong link between diabetes and erectile dysfunction, which affects about thirty million Western men at some point in their life. Although the problem is widespread worldwide, we seldom talk about it. With the introduction of Viagra, the issue has begun to come to light. This drug has become very popular, but in general it is much better to get to the root of the problem and try to rebalance the body.

Viagra helps increase libido, stamina, and endurance, and combats erectile dysfunction by increasing penile blood circulation, promoting a longer lasting erection.

However, problems have been reported in case of abuse, or in those suffering from hypertension. In any case there are a few natural alternatives to Viagra:

• **L-Arginine:** is an amino acid found in most protein foods that are animal-based such as chicken and beef, eggs and dairy products, but for better effects take it as a nutritional supplement. L-arginine increases blood flow to the penis and is safer than Viagra (it helps regulate blood pressure).

• **Siberian Ginseng** (*Eleutherococcus senticosus):* increases honey production for bees, enhances the development of sperm in bulls and secretion of milk in cows. It boosts energy drive for endurance.

• **Yerba Mate:** tea that comes from the bark of a tree (*Ilex paraguariensis*) from Paraguay. It is very rich in minerals and vitamin C. During times of great stress, it protects the adrenal glands that interfere with testosterone production. Ninety-seven percent of yerba mate contains caffeine only, but small traces act as vasodilators.

• **Yohimbé:** is one of the most effective natural remedies for erectile dysfunction. Yohimbé, or *Corynanthe yohimbi* grows in Zaire and Cameroon. Its bark contains substances that increase blood flow to the genital area, which promote a stronger and better erection and ejaculation. It also increases the body's sensitivity. But long-term use causes hypertension, headaches, anxiety, hot flashes, and heart attacks. In many countries, prescription is required to buy it in pharmacies. In the US, Holland, and other European countries it is sold in capsule or tea, but its use should always be carefully monitored.

• **Sarsaparilla** (*Smilax regelii*): Sarsaparilla has similar basic testosterone components, of which men with erectile difficulties are deficient.

• **Palmetto:** saw palmetto (*Serenoa repens*) is widely used to combat prostate disorders. It helps regulate hormonal stimulation of the prostate gland. It can be easily found in health food stores. Minimal side effects.

• **Taurine and stimulant drinks:** there are complementary products, such as drinks with taurine. Some are merely stimulants, like guarana. And many drinks with seductive promises usually contain caffeine in exaggerated amounts.

• **Oats:** simple and readily available, oats usually go unnoticed as an aphrodisiac. But they are a powerful regenerative food that has almost miraculous effects within a few days. The humble *Avena sativa* can be found packaged or as a drink ("milk" or **oat smoothie**), which becomes a mild and revitalizing aphrodisiac.

Blood flow enhancers

Increased blood flow to the penis is key to treating erection difficulties. There are nutrients and plants to enhance this flow, among which there is **ginkgo biloba**, taken as food supplement, 60 to 80 mg a day. There is also **coenzyme Q10**, which is an antioxidant that promotes energy production. And **vitamin E**, which further dilutes blood.

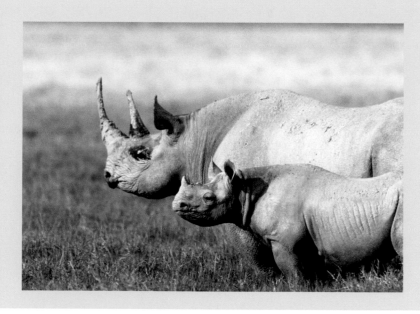

Love without nutritional deficiencies

Naturally, having a healthy heart and circulatory system is key for vitality and a powerful libido. To this end, **antioxidant vitamins C and E** protect arterial health. To avoid risks and maintain healthy vitamin levels, your diet should be rich in *citrus fruits, blueberries, berries, and melon. And avocados, nuts, seeds, and yeast.*

There are vitamins and minerals that are essential for healthy sexual activity. Let's review them, along with corresponding foods.

Iron. Essential for the production of vitamin C, for blood, and to give energy to our cells, and produce energy and activity (including sexual activity).
Red meat, liver, chicken, caviar, grapes, plums, apricots, egg yolks, whole grains, watercress, spinach, broccoli, beets, and beans.

Zinc. It is the most important and influential mineral in our sexual behavior and fertility. The tail of the sperm is made up of zinc, which gives it its peculiar driving capacity.

Zinc is essential for sperm production and has much to do with the health of semen (each ejaculation contains about 5 mg of zinc). At puberty, large amounts of zinc are needed for the development of the sexual organs, and it is essential for reproduction.
Seafood in general (especially oysters and sardines), eggs, cheese, lamb, chicken, turkey, liver, steaks, brown rice, lentils, squash, sesame seeds, spirulina, and whole grains.

Magnesium. Indispensable absorb calcium balance sex hormones and regulate heart muscle contraction and relaxation.

It is needed to produce energy, thus playing an important role in everything related to stamina, sensitivity, and sexual arousal as well as orgasm and ejaculation.
Vegetables and leafy greens, nuts, cheese, bananas, whole grains or flakes, grain seeds, (especially wheat germ), caviar, and seafood.

Calcium. Basic for heart and bones, calcium can revive tactile sensation in nerve transmission. It is needed for penile erection

(men) and the contraction of the labia and other sexual areas during an orgasm (women). It is a vital component of all body fluids.

Dairy, vegetables and leafy greens, beans, beets, watercress, prunes, nuts, dried fruit, seafood, and small fish such as sardines and whitebait.

Arginine. It is a basic amino acid and is derived from food protein. It is not only essential for all growth and sexual development, but it is also the main component of the head or "body" of sperm.
All animal-based foods, dairy, and popcorn (among plant-derived foods, popcorn contains the highest amount of arginine).

Chrome. Its deficiency affects the body's energy levels.
Soy and all its derivatives, yeast, cucumbers, onions, and garlic.

Selenium. It is essential to transform oxygen into energy and it is also related to the regulation of sexual activity, sperm production, and fertility.
All seafood, sesame seeds, and pumpkin seeds, Brazil nuts, and butter.

Iodine. The body needs it to produce thyroxine and stimulate the thyroid gland which regulates metabolic activity, energy

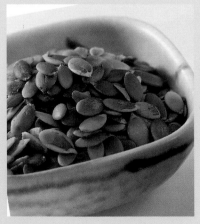

production and the formation of hormones. If the thyroid is not working well, you can experience a loss of sexual appetite.
Seafood in general, algae (particularly blue-green), spirulina, watercress, beets, turnips with leaves, fruit juices, watermelon, cucumber, tofu and spinach.

Coenzyme Q10. Also known as "ubiquinone." Each and every cell in our body needs this coenzyme so that our mitochondria (our little "power plants") produce and release energy we use at all times. Its production decreases with age, but the body always needs the same amount.
Spirulina, blue-green algae, chlorella and leafy greens (especially spinach), sardines, peanuts, and most animal-based foods.

Essential fatty acids. They are responsible for hormonal balance, nerve transmission, sensory responses, keeping skin in good condition and regulating fat storage in our body.
Omega-3s: *fish and shellfish, sesame seeds, pumpkin seeds and sunflower seeds, and their respective oils.*
Omega-6s: *avocados, squash, sunflower seeds, sesame seeds, flax seed and hemp, and their oils.*

Vitamin A is one of the main antioxidants, essential to cardiovascular health. Its two main sources are beta-carotene and retinol. Vitamin A is an important element for better sexual performance and health.
Beta-carotene-rich foods: *dark leafy greens (kale, Swiss chard, spinach, watercress, broccoli and parsley), and vegetables, yellow and orange fruits, both solid and juices (carrot, cantaloupe, peaches, and tomatoes).*
Foods rich in retinol: *milk, eggs, and fatty fish.*

B vitamins are very important for energy and digesting proteins and carbohydrates: **Vitamin B3** promotes greater flexibility of the capillary walls of the circulatory system, expanding them and allowing blood to circulate in a particular area (for example, the penis to initiate an erection). It does this by stimulating histamine (one of the hormones related to the body's immune system) which is needed during orgasm.

Vitamin B6 regulates the production and release of sex hormones and testosterone levels in men. It is usually quite common to find deficiency in men going through viropause.

Choline is not strictly a vitamin, but it is considered a B vitamin. It is a precursor to acetylcholine, the neurotransmitter of nerve impulses, so it is important to spread and boost energy levels and libido, resulting in a sense of wellbeing.
Whole grains (especially brown rice), legumes, nuts, yeast extract, meat, fish, eggs, dairy products, avocado, cream, mushrooms, cauliflower, and broccoli.

Vitamin C is essential for increasing the amount of semen and to ensure that sperm will flow freely. Vitamin C also has the ability to boost sexual activity and strengthen the sexual organs of both men and women.
Blackberries, blueberries, and cherries; citrus fruits, kiwi, mango, papaya, figs, potatoes, green peppers, broccoli, beets, and sprouts (e.g., soybean and alfalfa).

Vitamin E. It works in conjunction with Vitamin C and both are antioxidants. The internal protective nature of vitamin E is vital to ensuring health and vitality in all sexual activity.
All vegetables and leafy greens (broccoli, watercress, spinach, parsley, kale), avocado (huge amounts of vitamin E), brown rice, nuts and nutty oils, oats, and wheat germ.

Estrogen-related problems are a very common in the West, affecting fertility, the risk of ovarian and endometrial cancer, and a high percentage of breast cancer among women. For example, most food containers and wrappings have very similar properties to those of estrogens, which interfere with the delicate balance and function of progesterone and promote uncontrolled weight gain, fat reserves, and exacerbated PMS (Premenstrual syndrome).

Changes in menopause, or conditions such as vaginal dryness or hormonal changes during and after pregnancy often have adverse effects on libido. Luckily there are herbs and other nutrients that have traditionally served to treat all these disorders. And it seems that research today shows that these plants and nutrients are not just our grandma's recipes.

• **Evening primrose oil** (or starflower oil). The beneficial properties of *Oenothera biennis* oil for preventing and treating PMS are well known, although most important aspects reside in its qualities as a sexual activity enhancer. This valuable flower, from which the oil is extracted, is a rich source of GLA (gamma linolenic acid), an essential fatty acid for the production of sex hormones. Research has shown that decline in sexual activity due to fatigue generally improves with the use of evening primrose oil (or evening star, which is the same) and other essential fatty acids that help stimulate cell nutrient uptake.

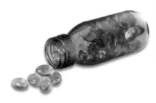

Evening primrose oil has great qualities as a stimulant of sexual activity.

Sesame seeds, sunflower and pumpkin seeds, nuts, and flaxseed are all excellent sources of essential fatty acids. It is always a good idea to include some of these health foods or oils in our daily diet.

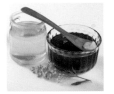

Royal jelly is an excellent tonic for the body and a sexual energy enhancer.

• **Bee pollen and royal jelly**. Both are an important source of essential fatty acids, carbohydrates, minerals, vitamins, and trace elements. Traditionally, pollen and royal jelly (a substance secreted by worker bees to feed the larvae, particularly those destined to become queen) are considered a great tonic for the human body, especially when energy is low due to stress or illness. Both are known to enhance sexual desire, and it is also said that pollen reduces hot flashes during menopause. Instead of consuming both substances on a regular basis, it is always better to take them during alternating periods of one or two months, with regular breaks in between.

• **Kombu seaweed**. No other known food contains greater amount of essential nutrients than kombu and blue-green seaweed. For a healthy and powerful "green concoction" just add it to milkshakes, smoothies, or sparingly in our favorite fruit juices.

• **Dong quai** *(Angelica sinensis)*. It is an adaptogenic containing compounds that are similar to estrogen and acts by lessening disorders related to increased estrogen in PMS. During menopause, it stimulates sexual appetite. Warnings: it can cause photosensi-tivity in some women, so avoid it if you have sensitive or very freckled skin.

• **Catuaba** *(Juniperus brasiliensis)*. This herb from Tupi, native land of the people of Brazil, is known for its sexual and erotic properties.

"Sexy" foods

Vitamins, minerals, and amino acids of many foods help boost sexual desire and overcome sexual problems. Strawberries, mangoes, oysters, pine nuts, and asparagus are the "top" sexy foods that will help us be our best selves in bed.

Corvina ♥♥♥♥	**Rye** ♥♥♥♥♥♥
Magnesium, essential omega-3 fatty acids, selenium, zinc.	Calcium, iron, magnesium, zinc, vitamin B and E.
Eggs ♥♥♥♥	**Spinach** ♥♥♥♥♥♥♥
Calcium, iron, zinc, vitamin B.	Beta-carotene, calcium, coenzyme Q $_{10}$, iron, magnesium, vitamin B and C.
Caviar ♥♥♥	**Tofu** ♥♥♥♥♥
Iron, magnesium, vitamin B (especially choline).	Calcium, iron, magnesium, phytoestrogens, vitamin A.
Popcorn ♥	**Pine nuts** ♥♥♥♥
Arginine.	Calcium, magnesium, zinc, vitamin B.

Originally it was used as an aphrodisiac. It acts as an adaptogen to relieve stress. It is also beneficial for men.

• **Phytoestrogens. Soybeans.** Phytoestrogens are estrogen like food found in very specific compounds that bind estrogen receptors of certain body tissues (and thus increases the total amount of estrogen circulating in the body). They are foods that can help reduce the risk of osteoporosis and enhance libido. Including: flaxseed, oats, sunflower seeds, pumpkin seeds, celery, barley, sesame seeds, poppy seeds, red onion, brown rice, red grapes, citrus, rye, peas, peppers, polenta, white beans, cherries, tomatoes, buckwheat, watermelon, garlic, and raspberries.

Soy products (soy isoflavones), are one of the most powerful medicinal food, a phytoestrogen success. Its origins are in Asia, and by way of our health food stores, it is increasingly becoming an essential food in the West.

Strawberries ♥♥♥♥♥
Beta-carotene, calcium, iron, magnesium, vitamin C and E.

Avocado ♥♥♥♥♥
Beta-carotene, essential fatty acids, iron, vitamin B and E.

Ginger ♥♥♥♥♥
Beta-carotene, calcium, iron, magnesium, zinc, vitamin C.

Mango ♥♥
Beta-carotene, vitamin C.

Squash ♥♥♥♥♥♥
Calcium, iron, magnesium, omega-3 and omega-6 essential fatty acids, vitamin B.

Almonds ♥♥♥♥♥♥
Calcium, magnesium, omega-3 and omega-6 essential fatty acids, zinc, vitamin B and E.

Shrimps and prawns
♥♥♥♥♥♥
Calcium, iodine, magnesium, phenylalanine, selenium, zinc.

Sesame seeds
♥♥♥♥♥♥♥
Calcium, iron, magnesium, omega-3 and omega-6 essential fatty acids, selenium, zinc, vitamin E.

Garlic ♥♥
Calcium, vitamin C.

Plums ♥♥
Calcium, iron.

Cream ♥♥♥
Arginine, calcium, vitamin B.

Celery ♥♥♥
Beta-carotene, selenium, B vitamins

Cheese ♥♥♥♥
Arginine, calcium, magnesium, zinc.

Brown rice ♥♥♥♥♥
Calcium, iron, magnesium, zinc, vitamin B

Papaya ♥♥♥♥
Beta-carotene, calcium, magnesium, vitamin C.

Tuna ♥♥♥♥
Omega-3 essential fatty acids, selenium, zinc, vitamin B.

Onions and leeks
♥♥♥♥
Beta-carotene, calcium, chromium, magnesium.

Figs ♥♥♥
Beta-carotene, calcium, vitamin C.

Lentils ♥♥♥♥♥
Calcium, manganese, magnesium, zinc, vitamin B.

Mushrooms and truffles
♥♥♥♥♥
Calcium, iron, magnesium, zinc, vitamin B.

Dark chocolate ♥♥♥
Magnesium, potassium.

Tomatoes ♥♥♥♥♥♥
Beta-carotene, calcium, magnesium, vitamin A, B and C.

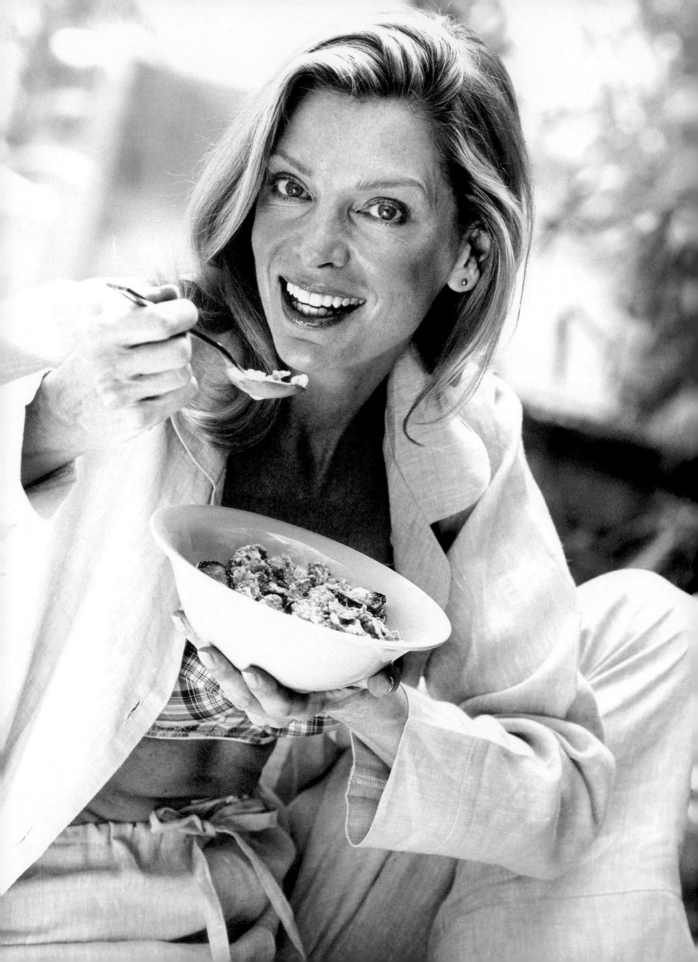

Age and food

2

The first months

After twelve months

After age five

Adolescence

Adulthood

Old age

Throughout life, diet varies greatly depending on the development of our bodies. As we know, we need to try to eat varied and well-balanced meals as much as possible to stay healthy and avoid disorders or diseases.

We have gathered here some dietary recommendations that ultimately depend on the condition, circumstances, and needs of each person. It is important to get to know your own body as much as possible, and make time to consult with a dietician from time to time. Some specialists are very good, they not only prescribe but most of all, they teach.

The first months

During the first four or six months, the baby must be fed only breast milk, which provides the necessary nutrients for a healthy development as well as substances that help build the child's immune and nervous system and protect him from digestive disorders, allergies, and infections. Besides being the best foundation for future development, strengthening the bond between a mother and child, breast milk is the most natural, comfortable, and affordable food for an infant.

Unfortunately, work prevents many mothers from spending time with their babies and breastfeeding is stopped prematurely (never before four months).

Formulas are the most common supplement, but they lack the beneficial properties found in mother's milk. They are usually made with cow, goat, or soy milk, and they take into account the baby's age and health. There are two types: "starting" formula (from birth to four or six months) and "continuing" formula (from six months on and until the baby is fed cow's milk).

When the baby is six months old you can introduce new foods, such as porridge and mashed grains, vegetables, fruits, and legumes. It is better not to introduce too many new foods suddenly and consult the pediatrician to get their opinion on when to start transitioning with the most appropriate food.

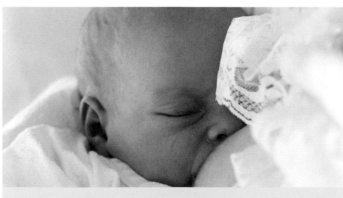

Breast milk allergy

It is estimated that two percent of babies born in Spain are allergic to their mother's milk, so they should be fed formula.

If the child rejects it, consult the pediatrician to examine the baby and prescribe the best type of formula.

The child should get the chance to get used to all the flavors and textures so he can enjoy a healthy and balanced diet. The greater the variety of foods they eat, the more their digestive capacity develops. Their possible reluctance to certain dishes (due possibly to allergies) must not change this goal.

As shown in the chart below, starting atnine months the child can have virtually the same meal program as the rest of the family, but with less fiber because an excess could impede the absorption of minerals such as iron and calcium, and a higher proportion of fats, since during this stage the child will consume between 1,100 and 1,300 calories a day and they need to absorb fat-soluble vitamins A, D, E, and K.

The World Health Organization recommends continued breastfeeding until 12 or 18 months.

After twelve months

When the child has their first birthday, they can eat almost the same food as the rest of the family: cow's milk, eggs, fruits, and vegetables, etc. After age two, their digestive system will have developed along with their first set of teeth; this allows them to eat even more different types of food. To prevent new food from causing digestive problems, give new food in very small amounts and wait a week or two until you are absolutely sure that the child is handling it well.

Their mealtimes have to match those of the rest of the family: three meals (breakfast, lunch, and dinner) and two snacks (mid-morning and afternoon). Continue this pace so that the child can develop healthy eating habits to ensure a continuous supply of energy.

CHILD'S EATING SCHEDULE

Younger than five or six months
Breastfeeding
Formula

At four to six months
Breastmilk
Gluten-free flours

At five or six months
Fresh juices

At six months
Soft vegetable purees
Fruit compotes

At seven months
Natural yogurt

At seven or eight months
Fresh cheese
Gluten flour
Thick vegetable purees
Crushed fruit

At nine months
Soft cheese
Egg yolk
Bread and cookies
Pasta or rice
Thin noodles

At twelve months
Cow's milk
Whole egg
Soft vegetable purees

At eighteen months
Whole vegetables

At age two
Cocoa
Nuts

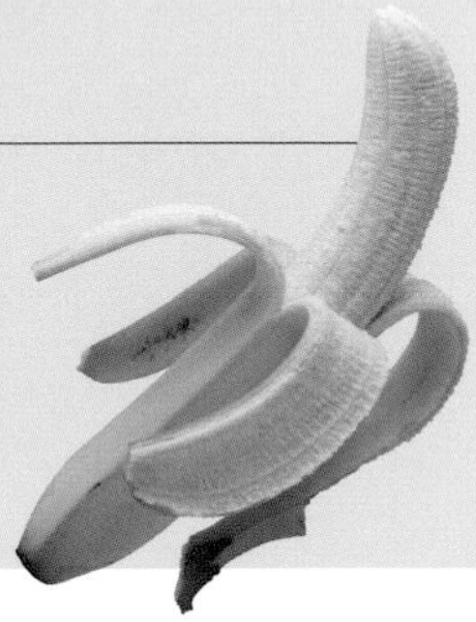

After age five

I t is typical for parents to comment on the high energy level that young children have. During this time, to a child the world is not only something new to discover, but their curiosity and ingenuity lead them to embark on adventures with unbridled passion.

Anything, however small and commonplace, grabs their attention and their activity can be frenetic. However, if there are no issues with hyperactivity (a problem that must be treated by a physician) parents should be patient and try to keep up with them as best they can.

Proper diet guarantees the energy supply the child needs.

This dynamism requires as much energy and nutrients as an adult, because not only do they need to replace the energy they burn, but the child also has to accumulate reserves to grow and develop properly and maintain a healthy weight.

After six months of age, children develop a sense of taste. They start to distinguish the differences between sweet and salty. A little later, before reaching one year of age, they begin to differentiate between bitter, spicy, sour, and tasteless. If during this training period the child only gets used to the two primary flavors, then they will reject all foods that are different and tend to eat only those that meet their expectations. So it is important to offer foods in a way that look appetizing. On the same plate, offer familiar foods along with new ones.

One of the most serious eating dangers is fast food ("junk food"). Its intense flavoring makes it very attractive for younger children, especially if you consider the flashy packaging and promotional gifts that are often included. Without outright forbidding it, we should not compromise: it is best to explain to children that they are not healthy.

School may pose some challenges to good eating habits instilled by the family because they may not match up with the cafeteria menu or with the eating habits of their classmates. The child may want to try their friend's favorite foods but if a different diet (vegetarian, for example) is followed at home, it is best to communicate with school administrators.

The child's diet is not much different from that of adults. Fruit (fresh and seasonal), vegetables, and whole grains instead of sweets and refined products. Vegetables, eggs, and dairy (especially yogurt) are the most important foods during this stage to ensure a balanced intake of protein, fats, and minerals (iron, zinc, and calcium).

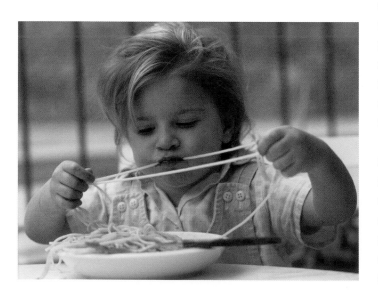

Adolescence

At age eleven, boys and girls begin to develop differently. In addition to continuing to grow, their body experiences changes related to the reproductive system, which requires certain dietary precautions. For example, a greater amount of energy: the nutritional needs of adolescents are much higher than those of their parents.

Physical development is coupled with a more defined personality and a desire for independence (at least with regard to their opinions), which can become contentious. Their eating habits will depend largely on those of their friends. During these years, teenagers begin to interact socially with much more freedom and often eat away from home. So, fast food becomes an easy and fun alternative to homemade food, which is often imposed on them and follows guidelines that they do not care for. But we must make them aware of the importance of healthy eating. Many teenagers are unaware that many problems experienced as adults (overweight, obesity, osteoporosis, or heart disease) are caused by poor nutrition during adolescence.

An unbalanced diet is the main reason our bodies lack phosphorus, calcium, and magnesium, which is necessary for bone development, and zinc, which is essential for the immune system.

Vitamins are important, especially B vitamins, which are present in eggs, dairy products, and certain fruits and vegetables, such as peppers, bananas, and potatoes. Although they may prefer to eat fries, soda, and well-seasoned meat, encourage them to eat eggs, whole grains, nuts, and legumes.

Recommended energy intake

Until age three	1100 to 1300 kcal per day
From age four to six	1400 to 1600 kcal per day
From age seven to ten	1700 to 2000 kcal per day

Recommended daily allowances

Carbohydrates	5
Fruits	3
Vegetables	3
Protein	2

Iron deficiencies

Women need a higher intake of iron than men because of blood loss during menstruation, which is especially abundant before the age of twenty, reducing iron levels ostensibly. The best way to compensate is to eat iron-rich foods every day, such as legumes and whole grains.

Servings recommended for adolescents

Oils and nuts	5
Grains and starches	5
Fruits	3
Dairy	4
Legumes	2
Vegetables	3

Anorexia and bulimia

These two eating disorders are, unfortunately, increasingly common among young men and women. The obsession with body image and their struggle to be accepted makes many girls and boys give too much importance to their appearance. Food becomes a way to control or change their body, and they tend to take drastic measures that can cause serious physical and psychological disorders that are potentially irreversible.

Although initially people suffering from these disorders were young upper-class women, for the past fifteen years there has been an increase in incidence among adolescents of both sexes (although lower in men) and in lower social classes.

Anorexia nervosa is characterized by an excessive obsession with weight loss. People who suffer from it develop a fat phobia and experience panic attacks when eating. Eating becomes a cumbersome process to get through as expeditiously as possible: selecting foods that provide fewer calories, doing plenty of exercise and, in extreme cases, inducing vomiting or taking laxatives and diuretics.

This eating disorder is not the cause of the disease, but its consequence. Much of the problem lies within the school and family environment, since in most cases it is all due to a troubled relationship with parents, friends, or classmates.

The duration of the disorder varies greatly, from a few months to a lifetime. To avoid it, raise awareness among teenagers of the importance of healthy eating and the attention our society gives to physical appearance. If there are deeper issues, then pay more attention and seek professional help. Intervene in the event that any of the following symptoms develop:

- **Obsession** with slimming diets.
- **Loss of appetite** or refusal of food.
- **Significant changes in body weight.**
- **Feelings of body shame.**
- **Irritability** and moodiness.
- **Frenzied activity** for no reason.
- **Dry skin** and brittle hair.
- **Hair loss.**
- **Menstrual disorders.**
- **Anxiety and confusion.**

From that moment on, the whole family must turn to the anorexic and put them in the hands of a specialized medical team, made up of doctors, psychologists, and dieticians. The treatment is long and slow (it can last from one to four years), it is not always effective, and relapses are common.

Bulimia is an eating disorder associated with anorexia, which compels a person to eat disproportionately when feeling anxious.

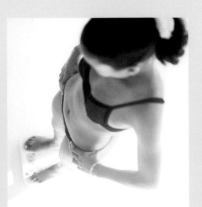

These crises can last an hour and lead to periods of depression in which the guilt, shame and contempt lead a person to decide to eliminate ingested food by means of induced vomiting, taking diuretics, or fasting. Symptoms commonly include:

- **Excessive concern** with body image.
- **Voracious and excessive eating** that usually occurs about three times a week.
- **Tendency to eat in secret.**
- Disruption of food with **vomiting.**
- **Severe abdominal pain.**
- Noticeable **fluctuations in weight.**
- **Binge eating** followed by periods of depression and self-loathing.

When any of these symptoms occur more frequently, we must put them in the hands of a team of specialists for therapy to control the disorder and heal. Keep in mind that bulimics hide their disease well, so we must pay close attention to their behavior and take action when necessary.

Adulthood

Our eating habits formed during childhood and adolescence affect our health as adults. However, this does not mean that after having been careful during the first twenty-five years of life you can forget about the next forty. . . .

Adulthood means special dietary needs related to work, where adults usually spend about half a day. Employment patterns in developed societies are increasingly similar, and that has meant eating anything (a sandwich and a soft drink) in the shortest time possible. Of course, this is not the most recommendable diet. It is even worse if this is done to continue working long hours, day after day. In addition, stress is an ever present problem in our society, and a poor diet only makes us suffer from stress earlier on.

Avoid eating at random hours throughout the day and try to combine home-cooked food (that gives you greater control over the quality of ingredients and its preparation) with snacks, or takeout. It is relatively easy to make small healthy and tasty changes. For example, make a salad and mix it with grains and protein (rice with vegetables and a couple of veggie burgers or sausages . . .)

Reduce fat intake (and completely eliminate animal fats) and have a regular supply of vitamins, minerals, and other nutrients. Dietary supplements are a good ally.

Diet and menopause

The production of estrogen during a woman's life is not uniform, but starting at puberty women experience an increase of estrogen that peaks between twenty and thirty years of age, and then begins to decrease until it is interrupted in their mid-forties. The end of this cycle is known as "menopause" and it is usually manifested as certain physical and psychological changes.

During this time, women often suffer from headaches, nausea, hot flashes, lack of energy, apathy, and irritability. Reduced levels of estrogen in the blood reduces physical strength and causes sudden exhaustion and osteoporosis.

To prevent a worsening of these symptoms and to rebalance the body, eat more calcium-rich foods (milk, yogurt, cheese) and essential fatty acids, as well as soy products, with pro-estrogenic qualities.

Also take the following precautions:

• **Control your weight.**
• Follow a **balanced diet** without animal fats.
• Make sure you are taking in enough **calcium** to avoid the risk of osteoporosis.
• Eat more **fruits and vegetables.**

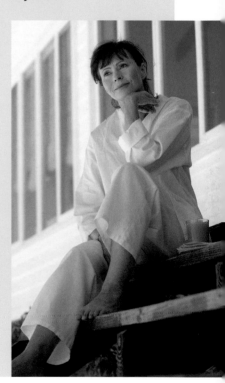

FOOD FOR WOMEN

Over time the female body experiences a series of changes that can only be addressed successfully through proper nutrition.

The hormonal system is much more important in women than in men because the production of estrogen and progesterone, which control menstruation, is regulated by the pituitary gland, which in turn depends on related emotional centers. Balance for women depends on diet, exercise, and surroundings that ensure their physical and psychological wellbeing.

From a dietary point of view, we must pay close attention to eating foods that are rich in folic acid (vegetables and grains), essential fatty acids, zinc, niacin, vitamin E, and "good" cholesterol.

FOOD FOR MEN

Starting at age twenty-five, one of the main problems experienced by men is overweight, something that does not really matter if it were not for the fact that excess fat tends to accumulate in the abdominal area, affecting the functioning of the digestive system, thereby increasing risk of intestinal toxemia: constipation, muscle aches, allergies, and digestive problems.

To avoid this, eat fewer protein-rich foods and saturated fats, in order to avoid risk of heart disease, diabetes, and colon cancer.

Men's bodies require a higher amount of protein, calories, vitamins (especially B vitamins), and minerals (including magnesium).

Sexual vitality depends not only on physical exercise and psychological balance: the type of food that is eaten also has an effect on it. Plant sterols and fatty acids from olive oil, as well as zinc, selenium, magnesium, and vitamin B_6, help regulate the production of sex hormones and maintain the quality of sperm.

Following a poor diet during adulthood aggravates the harmful effects of stress.

Old age

During the last stage of life the body experiences a decline in its capabilities. Its vital functions slow down and lose power. Its ability for regeneration is lower: bone tissue becomes less consistent, digestion becomes slower, and water loss will also increase. Therefore, we need to adopt various dietary changes that respond to these needs.

Just as in the previous stages, the dietary recommendations may be ultimately dependent on the physical and psychological state of each individual. Fewer calories are advised because the metabolism at this age is much slower than previously and there is less physical exercise.

The proportion of protein and fat should be less and of better quality.

Eat eggs, beans, and pureed vegetables for protein, and avoid fats in pastries and meats.

There should be more fiber in the diet since digestion usually slows down due to dental problems and salivation, and decreased peristalsis.

You have to moderate your intake of salt and sugar, as the risk of hypertension and diabetes is higher. As for dairy, nonfat yogurt can largely offset decalcification.

However, diet does not have to be bland and unvaried. Preparing food will require a little more imagination; for example, soups, casseroles, stews, and broths offset water losses (higher than in any other age group), while steamed food, papillotes, and purees, seasoned properly, enable more effective mastication.

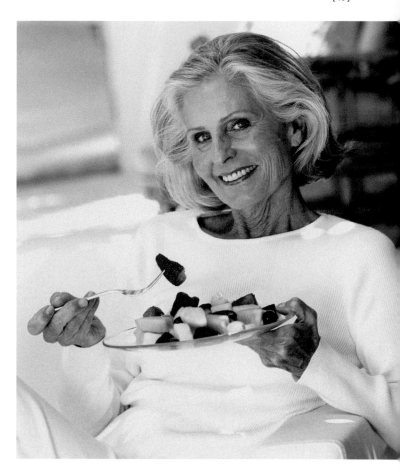

Most common disorders in old age

Disorder	Causes
Arthritis	Obesity, sedentary lifestyle, family history
Cancer	Bad habits (tobacco, alcohol), obesity, family history, high protein diet low in fruits and vegetables
Diabetes	Obesity, diet too rich in fats and sugars
Alzheimer's disease	Bad habits (tobacco, alcohol), high protein diet, low in fruits and vegetables, little intellectual exercise
Osteoporosis	Sedentary lifestyle, diet too high in protein and low in minerals
Cardiovascular problems	Bad habits (tobacco, alcohol), stress, obesity, diet too high in protein and low in fruits and vegetables

Old age brings new food needs to be covered in a more varied and tasty diet.

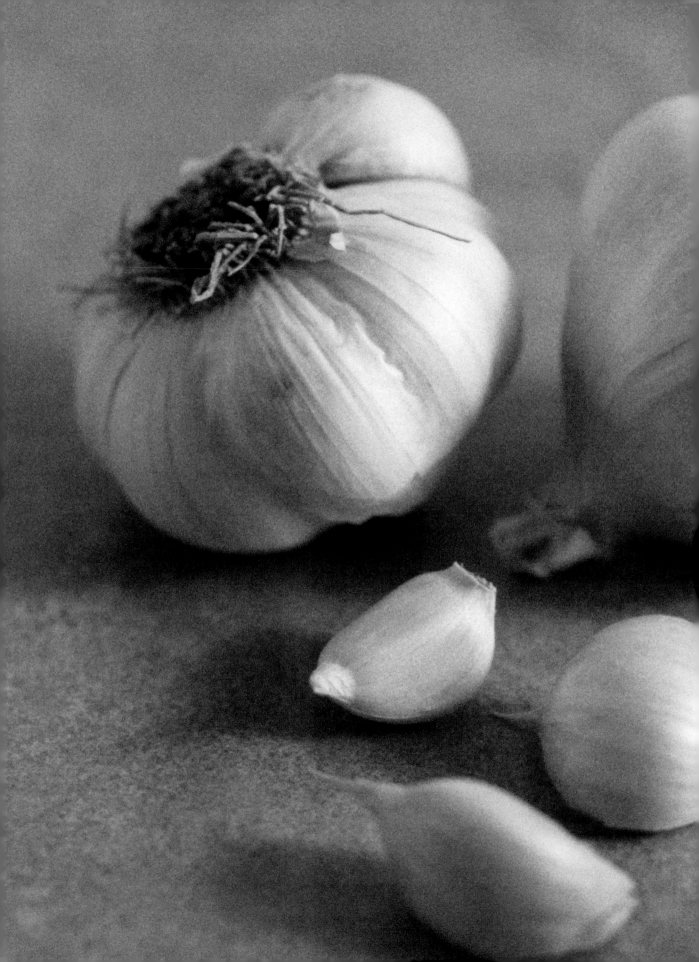

Superfoods

3 What to eat?

Choosing the best options

Types of additives

Nutraceuticals

Frozen food

GMOs

Irradiated food

Organic food

Superfoods

Food for hormonal problems

Food to prevent premature aging

Food to strengthen the joints

Food for healthy bones

Food for a healthy heart

What to eat?

"Ovarin, guaranteed fresh: not to be used after August 1, A.F. 632. Mammary gland extract: to be taken three times daily, before meals, with a little water. Placentin: 5cc to be injected intravenally every third day . . ."

In portraying the utopian society in *Brave New World* (1932), Aldous Huxley included passages like this to show the dangers of controlling life using science. In his classic novel, depression, anger, behavioral disorders, and other discomforts, however small, got a mandatory drug treatment.

Huxley's vision, which he countered years after with his ideal utopia (*Island*, 1962), may seem exaggerated. But only a few decades later (not seven centuries as he foresaw) all those visions are being met. And if you consider the increasingly generalized use of tranquilizers, sedatives, tonics, dieting pills, and other synthetic products that the chemical and pharmaceutical industry offers us today, we see how we depend more and more on artificial products to address issues caused by the pace of contemporary life.

The uses of chemical engineering and biotechnology are becoming ever wider. Genetically modified foods in markets around the world are controversial and this type of products will soon become available (even with dubious labeling) in supermarkets. According to some experts, they allow crops to multiply, resist pesticides, and their characteristics can be modified to make foods more "comfortable" (no pits, stackable shapes, uniform appearance, easy to transport . . . and a very long shelf life). But the potential harmful effects on the body have not been verified. Therefore be skeptical, or very wary of these products.

It is also possible to get concentrated nutritional compounds in capsules: well-known dietary supplements. Their nutritional value makes them a substitute for food in certain situations. As for nutraceuticals, in North America this term is used to designate food that meets the old adage "let your food be your medicine."

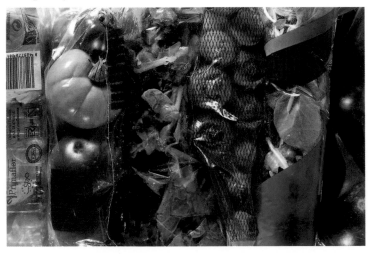

The appearance of GMOs has sparked controversy that will continue for some time.

As consumers, on the other hand, we hardly have time to pay attention to all the news related to these issues. If we also take into account that many new proposals are reviewed and the process is quite slow to ratify the new theories, there can be a lot of confusion. And yet, food is one vital aspect that cannot be neglected.

Every day, thousands of researchers in laboratories test whether food, raw or prepared in some way, protects against cardiovascular disease, alleviates joint pain, or helps boost the immune system. Moreover, if the human genome map is a vision of the future to help us determine whether we are more prone to certain types of cancer, is it naive to adopt a diet plan where natural antioxidant foods prevail?

We can enjoy good health and prevent many diseases and disorders through proper diet in which food, in addition to providing flavor and energy, helps us regulate and maintain our body.

As we can see, eating goes beyond simply replacing burnt energy.

Choosing the best options

Usually, when we go shopping we just grab what we need regardless of what we have at home. Much of the current food production uses various additives and treatments to preserve products. The pace of modern life often forces us to turn to packaged, pre-cooked, or frozen food. It is good to understand how these foods are made and what they contain in order to make better decisions.

FOODS WITH ADDITIVES

As good consumers, we should always read product labels. When it comes to food this issue is complicated because often times the ingredients list includes codes for dyes or preservatives, which we hardly know how to interpret.

What are additives?

Strictly speaking, a food additive is any substance not normally consumed as food itself or used as an ingredient in food (regardless of its nutritional value) as it is being processed.

By definition, additives are substances that are added to food in order to change its odor, color, taste or texture, improve its appearance, expedite growth, and extend shelf life. Food additives are quite numerous and are classified into different groups.

These additives may be natural or synthetic.

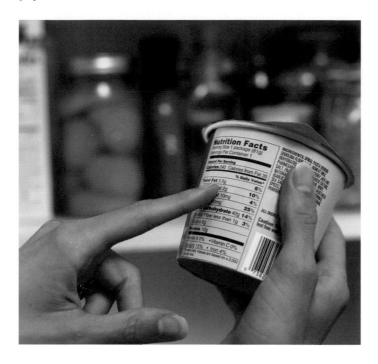

Each day there are increasing cases of food businesses breaking the law.

The former are much more expensive than the latter, so they are used at lesser rates. Their use is regulated and must meet three minimum requirements, namely:

• They should have an authorized and **suitable composition** for the purpose for which they are intended.

• **They should not have toxic substances** or contaminants outside the normal composition of foods.

• **The composition** and purity of food additives **cannot be altered**.

Legislation sets very precise rules for food businesses on the selection of raw materials, packaging, distribution, and storage of food.

However, each day more and more food companies are denounced by consumer organizations for breaking the rules. There are rare cases in which a particular product had little nutritional value and, instead, came with a host of additives to make it appetizing. There is no point hiding behind the alleged advantages of food technology: in these situations we can only speak of fraud. On the other hand, laws cannot regulate the way people live and eat in our modern societies: we eat too much, at the wrong time, too fast and we also eat products of dubious "quality" (i.e., excessively denatured).

We also need to keep in mind the risks that certain substances can pose for our health. Although the law prohibits using those that could be harmful in the short or long term, they are not all reliable. The safety of an additive depends not only on its chemical composition, but also on the proportion and frequency it is eaten. The ADI (Acceptable Daily Intake) sets forth the maximum amount of substances that our bodies can tolerate every day. Usually, it is expressed as a ratio of milligrams of additives per kilogram. Thus, an adult weighing 80 kg (176 lbs) can take 40 mg of potassium nitrite (ADI 5 mg per kilo of body weight) without any problems. However, this type of additive is responsible for carcinogens such as nitrosamines, so it is better to avoid foods that have it.

So, before blindly trusting the safety of additives, it is better to learn to differentiate them and act accordingly.

Types of additives

BULKING AGENTS
These are used to achieve the desired volume and texture in various products, such as sauces, butter, etc.

COATING OR MOLD RELEASE AGENTS
These are mostly waxes used to coat some foods (snacks, cheese, and citrus) or to separate them from their mold or container as in the case of candies, chewing gum, or industrial pastries. They also tend to use vegetable fats or oils.

FLOUR TREATMENT AGENTS
These are used to bleach flour, destroying existing carotenoids, and to improve it for kneading, as they modify its gluten structure. The process is similar to letting flour age naturally. In Spain these agents are not allowed for making bread.

MODIFIED STARCHES
These are used in ice cream, preserves, and thick sauces. In Spain they are used only in yogurt and canned vegetables. They are safe and completely harmless, although from a dietary point of view they provide the same calories as any other sugar.

ANTI-CAKING
They prevent sticking or clumping in substances such as table salt, powdered soups or sauces, and chemical yeast.

FLAVORINGS
As the name implies, enhances the flavor of food. Its purpose is commercial, since they make the product more palatable. Under current legislation, these additives just need to be listed with the generic term "natural flavoring" or "artificial flavor." Natural products are flavored with essential oils.

DYES
These are substances that "give life" to the product through an appetizing hue in soft drinks, liqueurs, puddings, pastries, and sweets.

Its use dates back to ancient times: Egyptians and Romans used to spice up their food with color, but the substances were completely natural: red was obtained from beets, orange from carrots, green from chlorophyll (from plant leaves) and ocher or brown came from clay soils. They not only used it to make food more appealing, but it also served to disguise when it was not in good condition.

Categories of food additives

Acidifying agents	Sweeteners	Flavor enhancers
Fillers	Emulsifiers	Emulsifying salts
Coating agents	Hardeners	Sequestrants
Flour treatment agents	Enzymes	
Modified starches	Thickeners	
Caking agents	Stabilizers	
Anti-foaming agents	Packaging gas	
Antioxidants	Propellant gas	
Dyes	Raising agents	
Preservatives	Gelling agents	
Acidity regulators	Wetting agents	

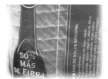

Under current legislation, coloring should not exceed that of fresh food, but you just need to walk around any supermarket to see that the reality is very different.

How can we know if a product has dyes? In principle, it should say so on the label. However, they are not always labeled individually and if they are, the nomenclature is so abstruse that we cannot make sense of it.

Today, natural and completely harmless dyes can be added without the need to specify them. In fact, food manufacturers are only required to indicate when dyes are used to improve product quality.

However, there is a group of dyes, known as "azo" whose use has caused serious controversy. For a time they were banned because after certain lab tests, it was concluded that they were carcinogenic. Subsequent studies showed otherwise and they were allowed for consumption once again. However, from a toxicological point of view, these additives are not recommended because although their carcinogenicity has not been demonstrated with certainty, it is clear that they can cause allergic reactions.

Besides dyes, the food industry uses color stabilizers, substances that lack coloring properties but which help stabilize the natural color of foods to keep them from changing.

PRESERVATIVES, ANTIOXIDANTS, AND ACIDIFYING AGENTS

Preservatives delay or prevent the growth of microorganisms such as fungi, bacteria, or mold that makes a product no longer edible. They can be applied to the surface of food or used as an ingredient. Its use is widespread in the food industry, but there are factors that must be taken into account:

• **People with asthma**, aspirin intolerance, or allergies should avoid food with benzoic acid or benzoates (E-210, E-211, E-213).

• **Nitrites** have a very high bactericidal action and are suitable for large amounts of meat products that are stored for long periods of time. Do not heat cured meat products (rich in nitrites) with foods rich in amines such as cheese to avoid carcinogenic nitrosamines from forming.

Potentially carcinogenic additives

E-210	Benzoic acid
E-211	Sodium benzoate
E-212	Potassium benzoate
E-213	Calcium benzoate
E-214	Ethyl parahydroxybenzoate
E-215	Sodium ethyl parahydroxybenzoate
E-216	Propyl parahydroxybenzoate
E-217	Sodium propyl parahydroxybenzoate
E-218	Methyl parahydroxybenzoate
E-219	Sodium methyl parahydroxybenzoate
E-239	Hexamentillentetramina
E-249	Potassium nitrite
E-250	Sodium nitrite
E-251	Sodium nitrate
E-252	Potassium nitrate

Vegetarians do not have that problem, but meat eaters should be careful with hot bacon and cheese sandwiches, pizza with pepperoni and cheese, ham and cheese sandwiches, etc.

• **Ascorbic acid and sorbates** have virtually no side effects.

• **White broths** have less sulfur dioxide than red broths, since sulfites act as color stabilizers. But be careful, because a couple of glasses meet IDA recommended levels for these preservatives.

• **Preservatives** designated as E-223, E-226, and E-227 destroy vitamin B1, and cause skin reactions in allergic individuals. Orange juice, pickled red cabbage, packaged salads, and packaged mashed potatoes contain these additives.

Antioxidants act similarly to preservatives: protecting foods from degradation by contact with oxygen, avoiding vitamin loss and fat rancidity. They can be obtained naturally or artificially. Acidifiers are the oldest known method for preserving food and as such they are essential ingredients in all canned preserves. Current legislation does not require that the label specify which type of acidifying agent is employed; it just needs to indicate "acidifying agent" or "acidity regulator." They usually do not pose any health risk, except sodium, potassium, and calcium sulfates, which may have laxative effect in high doses.

Most common preservatives

E-102	Tartrazine (lemon yellow)
E-104	Yellow quinoline
E-110	Yellow orange S, Sunset yellow FCF
E-122	Azorubine (red)
E-123	Amaranth (red)
E-124	Cochineal Red A, Ponceau 4R
E-127	Erythrosine (Pink)
E-131	Patent blue V
E-151	Brilliant Black BN
E-154	Brown FK
E-155	Brown HT

Natural dyes

E-120	Cochineal, carminic acid
E-160b	Bixin (orange)

SWEETENERS

They are used to make food sweeter. They can be natural or artificial, and they are distinctly much sweeter than sugar, but their caloric value is very low or nonexistent. Sugar substitutes do contribute calories but they do not require insulin to metabolize them, so diabetic people can take them without problem.

Saccharin is the most controversial of all sweeteners. It has been banned in some countries where it is considered a possible carcinogen. Like aspartame and cyclamate, it should not be used if you suffer from phenylalanine intolerance, as these substances may cause severe brain damage.

Diet or low calorie products include sugar substitutes as ingredients.

Using dyes to give an appetizing hue to foods is an ancient practice.

Most common preservatives

E-200	Sorbic acid
E-201	Sodium sorbate
E-202	Potassium sorbate
E-203	Calcium sorbate
E-210	Benzoic acid
E-211	Sodium benzoate
E-212	Potassium benzoate
E-213	Calcium benzoate
E-214	Ethyl parahydroxybenzoate
E-215	Sodium ethyl parahydroxybenzoate
E-216	Propyl parahydroxybenzoate
E-217	Sodium propyl parahydroxybenzoate
E-218	Methyl parahydroxybenzoate
E-219	Sodium methyl parahydroxybenzoate
E-220	Sulfur dioxide
E-221	Sodium sulfite
E-222	Sodium hydrogen sulfite
E-223	Sodium metabisulfite
E-224	Potassium metabisulphite
E-226	Calcium sulphite
E-227	Calcium bisulfite
E-228	Potassium bisulfite
E-239	Hexamentilentetramina
E-249	Potassium nitrite
E-250	Sodium nitrite
E-251	Sodium nitrate
E-252	Potassium nitrate

If the daily intake of these additives exceeds 50 g per day, it can cause diarrhea, vomiting, and stomach pains. Natural products use honey (make sure it is not heated after extraction), brown cane sugar, molasses, fruit syrup, or grains.

HARDENERS

Aluminum sulfates are usually added to candied and glazed fruit.

STABILIZERS

In this category, there are emulsifiers, thickeners, and gelling agents, which serve to homogenize prepared food. In general, these additives do not present major problems because they are either harmless or no side effects have been detected within recommended amounts. By law, it is not necessary to include stabilizers in the ingredients list.

The most common thickeners and gelling agents are fruit pectin, products derived from algae, flours or starches (including modified starches, which remain stable in heat and freezing temperatures) and gelatins. They are often added to dairy, pastries, instant soups, and creams.

The most common emulsifiers are egg yolk, soy lecithin, corn, or peanuts because they hardly alter the taste, texture, and color of pastries, chocolates, desserts, and yogurt.

WETTING AGENTS

Often used in baked goods, pastries, or candy that can become dry when stored for a long time. Two of which, sorbitol and mannitol, are sugar substitutes.

FLAVOR ENHANCERS

These enhance the flavor of all kinds of food, especially undercooled and dehydrated products. The most common is monosodium glutamate, a substance that in sensitive people can cause headaches, neck stiffness, and tightness in the temples.

POSSIBLE EFFECTS OF ADDITIVES

Azo dyes

- **Code.** E-102, E-104, E-110, E-120, E-122, E-123, E-124, E-127, E-128, E-129, E-133, E-151, E 154, E-155, E-160b, E-180.

- **Possible side effects.** Skin problems or allergic reactions in people sensitive to aspirin. Headache.

- **They can be found in . . .** Powders for making soft drinks, powders for making pastry products, powders for making instant soups, ice cream with artificial flavors, soft drinks, jams, sauces, cheeses, alcoholic drinks, canned fish, some cheeses, canned vegetables, canned fruits, and cookies.

Preservatives

- **Code.** E-210 to E-228 and nitrosamines (E-249 to E-252). E-1105 is harmful for those allergic to chicken eggs.

- **Possible side effects.** Allergic reactions, asthma, headaches.

- **They can be found in . . .** Canned vegetables, canned fish, canned fruit, dried fruit, jam, orange juice, margarine, mayonnaise, broth, banana peel, citrus peel, dairy products, some cured cheeses, provolone, cured meat, sliced bread, dehydrated mashed potatoes, industrial baked goods, and caviar.

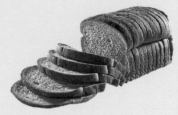

Antioxidants

- **Code.** E-310 to E-312. E-320, E-321.

- **Possible side effects.** E-310 to E-312, stomach aches. They are harmful to asthmatics or those who are hypersensitive to aspirin. E-320 and E-321 increase cholesterol level in the blood; they are not recommended for infants and young children.

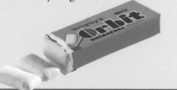

- **They can be found in . . .** Breakfast cereals, cookies, nuts, candies, powders to prepare instant mashed potatoes, flavored rice, vegetable fat, and gum.

Sweeteners

- **Code.** E-951 (aspartame), E-952 (cyclamate), and E-954 (saccharin).

- **Possible side effects.** The first two can cause disturbances in people with phenylketonuria. Saccharin is a controversial substance. In some countries it is prohibited because it is considered carcinogenic. In Spain its use is authorized.

Flavor enhancers

- **Code.** E-620 to E-625.

- **Possible side effects.** They can cause headache, neck stiffness, and tightness in the temples.Not recommended for young children.

- **They can be found in . . .** Soups and prepared sauces, meat and fish concentrates, and certain yeasts.

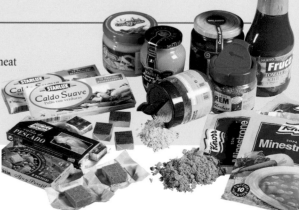

Nutraceuticals

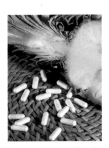

Nutraceuticals mark the era of fast and easy prevention.

In many science fiction movies with robots, futuristic costumes, and computers, the characters eat their food in capsules. Although it may seem a little strange, this solution is not as crazy as it sounds, because these foods, called "nutraceuticals" are already here. They are not exactly like the movies (no pizza pills); rather, they contain dehydrated or plant extracts. Once scientists announce the discovery of any substance that helps to lower cholesterol or fight cancer, then such substance begins to gain a lot of popularity. For now, we can find extracts with therapeutic properties of certain plants, vegetables, and fruits in natural health food stores. So instead of going to the market to choose the best vegetables of the day, you can go to the health food store and buy a bottle of carrot tablets and ingest its active ingredients. There are also papaya, artichoke, or garlic capsules or pills with the equivalent of four cups of green tea. As we said: food in pill form.

Nutraceuticals mark the era of easy and fast prevention, if we do not want to bother peeling fruit or washing vegetables, or having our hands smell like onion. These capsules tend to contain high concentrations of active components, for example garlic, which we need to consume in large quantities during an illness; this is an impossible task for many, but it is quickly solved with a few garlic capsules a day.

Everything indicates that it is time for us to grow any vegetable substance that is beneficial to our health, and then have it extracted and packaged into easy to swallow tablets. However, where the makers of dietary supplements see a straight line from growing vegetables all the way to production of the tablet containing its essence, some food experts see a winding road full of ups and downs.

When we read that there are lower rates of breast cancer among Asian women than among Westerners, we begin to have our doubts: Is it due to diet? Is soy or green tea responsible? Does food combination matter?

Many researchers have tried to find answers by isolating the compounds that seem to prevent the development of diseases. Such a task is not easy, as it requires endless analysis and time-consuming tests. Sometimes it is difficult to know with certainty whether an active component is still good after processing it. And if it does, there is no assurance that the effects of ingesting it along with other substances are the same as when taken alone. Regardless, it is important to consider the integrity of the plants, as explained by Mikel Iturrioz Garcia, technical director of Solgar, subsidiary of an American company that since 1947 produces all kinds of vitamins and nutritional supplements:

"A plant's whole therapeutic capacity is never only on one isolated active ingredient. We should never separate ourselves from nature, from the plant itself. "

However, and despite the reservations that we might have regarding these products, many food experts have faith in them. There are multiple naturopaths that recommend them. Moreover, although broccoli and Brussels sprouts contain six of the most potent anticancer agents, most people do not usually include them in their daily diet. Perhaps taking them as nutraceuticals would solve this problem.

The question is: Should we give nutraceuticals a try? Obviously, enjoying the taste of a juicy pineapple is not the same as taking it in a capsule, but if you suffer from digestive disorders, then bromelain (a powerful enzyme capable of digesting some 1,000 times its weight in protein and which is at the heart of the fruit) can alleviate your symptoms if you take several capsules daily.

Keep in mind that despite providing the body with a significant proportion of therapeutic ingredients, nutraceuticals must always be considered a supplement, as they fail to meet our daily needs of fiber, vitamins, and minerals.

Before buying them, talk to your doctor about which ones are best for your individual needs and always read the label carefully. It is essential to ensure that the products are organic and are not about to expire.

A new food era is just beginning, and we must take certain precautions. Currently, variety is much less than expected. However, ongoing research projects will gradually cover the entire spectrum of prevention.

Below, you will find the top ten most effective nutraceuticals. They are a must for those who think of food as a tool for developing all our physical and spiritual strengths.

GARLIC

It seems incredible that a single food is capable of reducing cholesterol levels in the blood, lower blood pressure, boost the immune system, and reduce cancer risk. Or at least that's the contention of the majority of the scientific community.

Many findings on the medicinal properties of garlic are based on the study of natural garlic extracts. However, laboratory tests have yielded spectacular results when very high doses were administered. The optimum percentage is about 2.5% of the amount of food eaten within a day, which is equal to a lot of heads of garlic. But taking it does not have to be hard: garlic can be had in concentrated form as capsules or extracts.

BROCCOLI

As mentioned before, it seems that broccoli is one of the most effective vegetables to prevent the risk of cancer. Its secret lies in sulforaphane, a substance that protects DNA strands and prevents the appearance of tumors.

The tablets contain 500 mg broccoli extract, of which 200 mg corresponds to sulforaphane, an equivalent amount obtained from a normal serving of this crucifer.

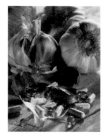

Garlic lowers cholesterol, lowers blood pressure, stimulates the immune system, and reduces the risk of cancer.

ONION

Many specialists consider it as healthy as garlic because their virtues are very similar. However, few people like to eat it raw. One of its main active components, allyl propyl disulfide, is very beneficial for health, although it is best known for its thiopropionic acid (its volatile essence), which is responsible for making us cry when we cut it. To prevent or treat diseases of varying severity, we need to ingest large quantities (as with garlic), so one option is to have tablets made from its dried and crushed bulbs.

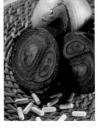

Onion is therapeutic when ingested in large amounts, so tablets could be a good choice.

PAPAYA

This delicious tropical fruit is rich in enzymes such as papain and chimopapain, plus vitamins A, B, and C. In tropical countries, where it originated, it is consumed as an aperitif, a digestive, and intestinal regulator. Regarding the tablets, it is possible to find them made from pulp, leaves, and fruit, and its active ingredient: papain. Taking 0.1 to 0.5 g relieves digestive disorders and gastric and duodenal inadequacies.

CAYENNE PEPPER

Capsaicin, which is responsible for the burning sensation that hot peppers give, appears to neutralize carcinogens found in some foods. Its power is such that it is even considered capable of disabling those in tobacco smoke. Supplements are simply filled with cayenne and they are a valid alternative if you prefer foods that are not too spicy. Another invaluable aid provided by the capsaicin is its action against joint pain, although in this case the spicy substance is mixed with a cream and applied to the affected area.

PINEAPPLE

The tablets of this fruit are powerful bromelain concentrate, an enzyme that alleviates digestion problems and constipation, and which works remarkably well in the treatment of phlebitis, atherosclerosis, and arthritis. In addition, it is believed that the active substance induces a chemical-physiological reaction that helps dissolve cellulite nodules and works well for slimming down.

MUSHROOMS

In China and Japan certain native species are used to boost the immune system. They are rich in phytonutrients: polysaccharides, triterpenes, phytosterols, and lignins. Studies on the stunning effects of these mushrooms were so great that we can now take capsules made from shiitake, maitake, and reishi mushrooms to benefit from their properties.

SOY

This oriental vegetable has been completely adapted to our diet and it provides a lot of protein.

Many studies have shown that taking soy protein powder daily reduces cholesterol by up to 34%. It is also believed that isoflavones (estrogen-like chemicals found in soy) can reduce the risk of breast cancer and prevent the development of malignant tumors. In addition, they help support strong bones and relieve swelling.

There are many ways to eat soy: green beans (used often in veggie burgers or meatballs), tofu (or soy "cheese"), tempeh (fermented soybeans), "milk," flour, lecithin, miso (fermented paste), tamari (seasoning), etc. As if this were not enough, there are also soybean extract tablets or soybean powder, although these do not contain fiber and carbohydrates, they do have active ingredients and can be added to various other foods, such as scrambled eggs, soup, or breakfast cereal.

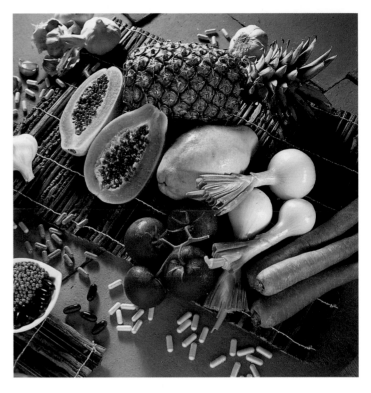

TOMATO

Some years ago, tomatoes appeared in newspaper headlines around the world thanks to a researcher at Harvard University, Edward Giovannucci, who explained the advantages of a solution based on Neapolitan sauce, pizza, and cooked tomatoes to prevent various types of cancer, especially prostate cancer. According to this scientist, this effect is due to lycopene, an antioxidant abundant in red tomatoes.

A tablet of 5,000 mg of lycopene has this substance extracted from tomato seeds. Although Giovannucci's research aimed to study the effects of tomato itself, it was concluded that lycopene is what gives the tomato its ability to reduce the risk of cancer, although it is possible that other components influence the process.

CARROT

Throughout this book, we see the many properties that this vegetable has. Tablets allow eating it in dehydrated form. Carotenes and vitamin E protect from oxidation and prevent external and progressive loss of skin elasticity. But it also contains provitamin A and it is considered one of the best dietary supplements to protect our eyesight.

Nutraceuticals may be the most effective way to prevent deficiencies in our bodies.

Frozen food

Not long ago when I participated in a Japanese cooking class, a colleague commented that it is possible to live without a fridge, and as proof he mentioned his grandmother, who lived in a village in Portugal where she used a "crisper."

With the pace of life that we have set for ourselves, refrigerators have become indispensable. And if these appliances are needed, what about frozen food? A few decades ago, the freezer was seen as a tool for saving considerable time: we could prepare several dishes and freeze them to consume days later.

Soon after, there came frozen meals and fruits, to facilitate the work of those lacking time, desire or cooking experience. However, are frozen products as good as fresh foods? Are they reliable? Before answering hastily, we should make some clarifications.

Frozen food that we prepare at home is not the same as precooked frozen meals, since the latter usually includes unhealthy additives.

Freezing itself stops or reduces biological degradation, microorganisms do not reproduce at low temperatures, but yet they do not disappear. When thawing food, bacteria go back into action, so you have to cook food right away.

Despite its usefulness, take into account that freezing lowers nutritional content of fruits and vegetables. In most cases vitamins C and E, pantothenic acid and pyridoxine (vitamin B6), and other B complex are lost. If they are also blanched before freezing, we find that a significant proportion of water-soluble vitamins are lost.

The cellular structure of plant and animal-based foods is not harmless, because freezing tends to alter and, in some cases, destroy tissue, with a consequent loss of nutrients. As the temperature drops, tissue cells undergo a process of expansion that mixes previously separated substances resulting in chemical reactions that affect the organoleptic characteristics, the product's texture or its nutrients, and different pigmentation appears in natural products which are sometimes concealed with dyes.

Tips for using frozen food

• Use them only sparingly.
• Avoid elaborate dishes with vegetables or combinations that may have additive (patties, breaded, pizzas, stews, paellas, and so on).
• Pay attention to the expiration date.
• Food should be cooked or eaten as soon as it thaws.
• Defrosted food cannot be refrozen.
• Frozen food must stay cold at all times: from the place of purchase to the home freezer.

In fact, change in taste and odor is due to reactions produced by oxidizing or hydrolyzing enzymes that alter fatty compounds in vegetables. Discoloration in frozen fruit and vegetables, however, is due to the degradation of chlorophylls, carotenoids, anthocyanins, and other natural pigments.

On the other hand, it is possible to buy frozen vegetables without additives. Cabbage in all its varieties, onions, garlic, peas, green beans, chard, and spinach resist quite well. However, when paired with other ingredients such as potatoes, rice, creams, etc., additives have to be added. The best thing to do in these cases is to read the labels. Additive charts will be very useful to determine which are the most deleterious additives. However, keep in mind that some products, such as potatoes for frying or salads, have such few additives that they are not listed in the ingredients.

To avoid confusion, follow this rule: the more elaborate the dish, the more likely it contains additives.

Besides all these precautions, frozen foods must be kept cold. The time between the purchase of the product and placing it in the freezer should be minimal. For this reason, some companies have specialized in transporting food in specially equipped trucks.

Many nutrition experts believe it is preferable to eat small portions of food that is fresh rather than big and elaborate meals. But what can we do when there is not enough time to cook? It is all a matter of organization. We can prepare food at home and keep it in the freezer, and we can make something simpler but no less nutritious. The daily salad that experts recommend does not take long to make. Food is a good way to express our love. Frozen foods are too impersonal.

GMOs

Advanced science applied to foods results in genetically engineered or "transgenic" food.

A few years ago, the very thought that you could get a tomato to last longer, without seeds, or have their color, shape, and size identical throughout the crop seemed more like science fiction than reality. Nowadays, it is possible to buy an ear of transgenic corn in a grocery store.

WHAT ARE GMOS?

They are microorganisms, plants, or animals that have been modified by genetic engineering techniques to change their DNA structure. This disorder usually involves removing a gene or adding genes of a different vegetable or animal organism to give it a new characteristic.

Some plant species have been treated to resist certain parasites or insecticides. The acronym that identifies them as such is GMOs (Genetically Modified Organisms).

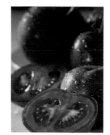

Genetically modified foods are the latest standard of scientific advances applied to food.

WHAT ARE THE ADVANTAGES OR UNCERTAINTIES?

Multinational corporations and public research laboratories that developed this new technique argue that the main advantages are increasing the quality and quantity of agricultural production and environmental protection. However, its benefits are not very clear and there are many groups that reject using GMOs and question health and environmental problems that may develop over the short and long term, while, on the other hand, there are concerns with the future and independence of farmers.

Keep in mind that chronic toxicological tests for this new generation of foodstuffs have not yet been made. Does this mean that we are all involved in a scientific experiment whose consequences are unknown?

The main problem is that there is little chance for follow-up, so that leaves room for mistakes that can be irreversible. For gene therapy, patients are volunteers and they undergo medical observation. But with GMOs there is no one to assist us.

G. E. Seralini, researcher at the Laboratory of Biochemistry and Molecular Biology at the University of Caen in France, said this about GMOs: "One day, the chairmen and members of committees should publicly respond to the scientific quality of the reports which gave a favorable opinion for their distribution. If they were to disseminate toxicological evaluations of GMOs, which have resulted in decisions for marketing in Europe, the scientific community would smile bitterly at the sight of the three cows or ten treated rats, of which we have incomplete short term experiments."

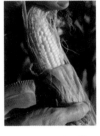

Plants like corn have been specially engineered to resist herbicides.

GROWING GMO CROPS

There are plants, such as corn, soybeans, and cotton, that have been specially engineered to resist herbicides. Their makers claim that it is a great advantage for the farmer, who can apply antiparasitic products without fearing for their crops.

Although GMOs are supposed to require fewer applications of chemicals, they require an increase in herbicide use (as has been shown with Monsanto's Round Up) in regions where transgenic crops have been introduced. For example, in Argentina, its use has tripled in three years, from 5.2 million to 15.8 million gallons (twenty million to sixty million liters). As if that were not enough, we must bear in mind that plants soaked in herbicides are used as animal feed. There are other plants, known as Bt, that are resistant to certain insects, such as corn borers, which produce insecticidal toxins in all their cells along the vegetative cycle. Furthermore, cross-pollination between transgenic and non-transgenic plants causes uncontrollable contamination, as it was recently seen in France.

WHAT ABOUT THE FARMERS?

What about the farmer who does not want to grow GMO varieties? And what about the organic grower who can lose the organic farming labeling, and have no possibility of appeal?

Historically, farmers produced their own seeds; only recently, with the emergence of hybrid crops, have they been forced to buy seeds each year. However, more than one billion people still rely on seed produced in the farm itself and biotech

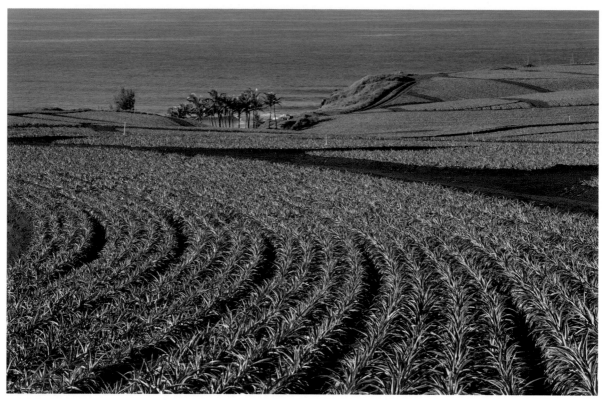

Although it is believed that GMOs require less chemical applications, herbicide use is increasing.

multinationals are trying to take this right away from farmers. Each genetically engineered seed is patented and farmers who use them have no right to replant the harvested product. What does this mean? It means that each year you have to pay royalties to multinationals.

Public research is largely geared toward biotechnology, and delay in researching GMOs is also detrimental to organic agricultural practices.

AN IMPERFECT FUTURE

Controversy surrounding GMOs is part of the great album of eugenics, which has been getting longer for some time: cloning,

mapping the human genome . . . However, can eating genetically modified foods be considered progress? Why is it that we cannot assert what their effects will be in the medium- to long-term? If they are not beneficial, are they at least safe? Do they improve our immune system or prolong our life? There are too many unanswered questions.

For these reasons, environmental organizations worldwide are organizing campaigns calling for an immediate and complete moratorium on the marketing and cultivation of GMOs, banning patents on living organisms, developing public research on alternative methods of agriculture.

Irradiated food

It is not often that we hear about this type of food even though it has existed for many years. To define them, we can say that they are foods that have been subjected to doses of ionizing radiation so they can be stored longer.

A LITTLE HISTORY

Although this technique had some impact in the press a few years ago, it actually began back in the early twentieth century. In 1916, one of the first tests was conducted in Switzerland. Yet it was not until 1953 that the method was first developed in the United States under the program "Atoms for Peace," which aimed to use nuclear technology for civilian use. Four years later, it was used in Germany for the first time by applying radioactivity to spices used in sausages. The Soviet Union was the first government to allow food irradiation in 1958. Since then, more than thirty countries have allowed irradiation in 28 different types of food for human consumption. Currently the main countries using this technique are China, South Africa, and some countries in the former Soviet Union.

WHAT DOES IT CONSIST OF?

Food exposure to radiation aims to increase its shelf life.

To irradiate food, permanent facilities are used, although models were also developed that can be used in field crops or large fishing boats.

The radiation sources used are mainly cobalt 60 and cesium 137, which are both radioactive waste from nuclear power plants. X-rays are also used with certain precautions to avoid exceeding allowed radiation limits. Radiation doses vary: while the Codex Alimentarius caps its limit at 10 MeV (million electron volts), the Food and Drug Administration (FDA) recommends not exceeding 1 meV. To get a better idea, this means multiplying the radioactivity used for an x-ray by ten or a hundred million. Despite its magnitude, the limit is safe, as food becomes radioactive only above 10 meV.

DIFFERENT METHODS OF RADIATION

Different effects are achieved depending on the radiation level to which food is subjected.

• **Radiorization.** Foods are subjected to low doses of radiation. This keeps potatoes and onions from sprouting, fruit from rotting, and helps stored grains to resist pests.

• **Radicidation.** With medium doses of radiation, the number of microorganisms that break down food (yeasts, mold, and bacteria) is reduced, extending shelf life and reducing risk of food poisoning, as with salmonella.

What happens to food when it is irradiated?

Damage occurs to most vitamins, especially A, C, D, E, and K as well as to some B vitamins; especially B1, which is rapidly destroyed during storage. Vitamin E disappears completely, even if it is added afterward. This is extremely important in foods like fruits and vegetables, as they are the main source of vitamins in many diets. Vitamins are also lost by irradiation because shelf-life is lengthened and then food has to be cooked.

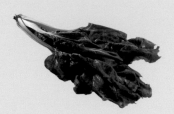

Taste and texture of food (especially fish, meat, oils, and fats) is altered in addition to its chemical structure, to the extent that new chemical compounds known as radiolytics are created. Some are similar to those that appear when a food is simply cooked, but others are specific to radiation such as benzene, formaldehyde, and other known mutagenic and carcinogenic compounds. The amount of radiolytics that appear depends on the level of radiation to which food has been exposed, and in many cases there is no way to ensure that radiation was conducted within the established control limits.

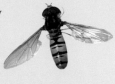

Mutations may occur in insects, bacteria, and viruses that are to be eradicated. To make matters worse, radiation not only eliminates toxins produced by bacteria (aflatoxins), but it can increase its production and while it is true that it eliminates yeasts, mold, and other microorganisms responsible for bad odors, it also prevents detection of spoiled food.

Irradiation can be used to eliminate other measures: some foods that do not meet food safety regulations are irradiated and then offered for sale.

• **Radappertization.** Higher radiation levels are used to completely sterilize food. If meat is subjected to this process, it can be kept almost indefinitely.

This type of food irradiation has other benefits for the food industry. It increases the baking quality of wheat flour, allowing it to mix with soy flour; it gives antioxidant properties to sugar (which may replace other additives); increases the amount of juice that gets extracted from grapes; and "ages" broths and spirits, etc.

THE EFFECTS

Proponents of irradiation argue that this system of conservation extends the shelf life of food without resorting to preservatives, colorings, and other additives. Such a statement is not entirely accurate, because irradiation has negative effects on food that can only be remedied with the use of substances that are applied before and after subjecting the product to radiation. To make matters worse, it does not replace other preservation methods because oftentimes in addition to being irradiated, food has to be frozen.

IRRADIATED FOOD LABELING

In Europe, since 1979 there is a directive requiring labels that explain any processes that a food product has undergone, including irradiation. But it does not apply to products that are sold in bulk, such as fresh fruits and vegetables.

As for irradiated food labels, it is also expected that they bear an identifying symbol, disclose any nutritional losses and give a date to indicate the age of the product, as these types of foods can look fresh for a long time.

WHY IS FOOD IRRADIATED?

Food irradiation, far from being a solution to problems with conservation, is one more method among the many that exist. But is it safe? It would appear that if the European Union has forced its members to authorize its use, it does not represent serious problems for human health. However, as we have seen, it is a method that can be used to "mask" natural processes of food. We should not forget that it can also be tied to other systems of conservation or improvement, so the end result is no less a denatured food. Doesn't it seem as though irradiation has more to do with the food industry's need to store food for longer periods and transport it for longer distances (avoiding losses) than with consumer needs? Let's not forget the origins of this technique, which is not exactly the food industry but the nuclear industry, which would mean a solution to the problem of how to recyclenuclear waste. In fact, 36% of the IAEA (International Atomic Energy Authority) budget is intended for research into using nuclear energy in food and agriculture, besides trying to convince the scientific community of the goodness of food irradiation.

Organic food

Organic products are balanced and rich in nutrients when grown without agrochemical products and respecting nature's rhythms.

With so many low-quality (and therefore low-price) products in the market, it is difficult to speak of wonderful foods unless they have the "organic" label to absolve them of any suspicion. But does this mean that good quality food must be organic?

IN DEFENSE OF ORGANIC PRODUCTS

We could start by saying that organically grown produce yields healthy animals, fresh foods that retain their natural properties, and they also do not abuse the environment or the farmer because organically grown animals, fruits, and vegetables do not have artificial fertilizers, nor hundreds of insecticides, pesticides, fungicides, herbicides, waxes, hormones, antibiotics, and other additives. However, some organic food may be exposed to pollution (by inorganic waste found in water, soil, and air) or other pesticides used in neighboring farms.

Unlike soils that have undergone chemical abuse, organic soils are biologically rich, and well balanced with natural microorganisms and bacteria. Compost, as a basis for fertilization, makes soil the perfect setting to feed microorganisms that live in it. Chemical fertilizers kill microbial life in the soil. The difference is remarkable, since organic products have a higher proportion of nutrients, whereas all industrially engineered products contribute toxins.

Moreover, there is another ecological element at play: every time an organic food is purchased, it helps the planet's biodiversity and prevents death of plants, birds, useful insects, small mammals, etc. Conventional farming uses many products to kill all kinds of organisms that can harm the development of the plant, from insects to weeds. These chemicals are not safe, even in small doses. Neither are their long-term effects good for our fields and our bodies.

With regard to pesticide residues in vegetables, recent reports from the European Union indicate that about 36% of produce contains pesticides and that 2% exceed the maximum limits allowed. In Spain in particular, fruits have up to 60% (with orange and peach as the most polluted), followed by vegetables, with 26% and grains, with 15% (rice has higher rates).

Obviously, meat is not safe because the animals also consume foods with toxins. If they are given hormones, dioxins, antibiotics, and other drugs, the result can be terrible.

As if that were not enough, it's no secret how animals intended for consumption are kept: malnourished and crammed in appalling conditions. Why do we tolerate such abuse? Why do we eat animals that are stressed and sick? Perhaps we need to think about our own responsibility in that process.

Meat eaters have the option of buying organic meat of animals that are fed "good old fashioned" grain, seeds, and other organic feed, whereby their metabolism is not altered. And this is not limited to eating meat: ovolactovegetarians should note that yogurt, milk, eggs, or cheese can also come from an animal raised in one way or another depending on whether the products are organic or not. As mentioned earlier, the best solution is to check for an "organic" label guarantee.

Be careful with grains!

Whole grains are highly recommended for fiber and minerals, and should be organically grown. Those that have been cultivated by the agrochemical industry carry pesticides in greater proportion and are more dangerous.

Whenever you purchase an organicproduct you obtain a greater amount of nutrients and you help maintain the planet's biodiversity.

In Spain there is a Regulatory Board for Ecological Agriculture (CRAE) and each region has its share of responsibility. In the rest of Europe there are agencies to support and guarantee the quality of organic products.

They can help you determine when foods are produced in accordance with strict criteria that do not allow for artificial substances and respect natural cycles, without synthetics.

What about water?

This element that is so essential to life is also affected by agrochemicals because some fertilizers and chemicals come from land cultivated with inorganic products and move through rivers, lakes, wells, streams, or groundwater and inevitably come out through the tap.

BEST FOR OUR HEALTH AND THE PLANET

Today, there are people who care about changing how some sectors of the industry mistreat the land and animals. Perhaps the main objection to abandoning industrial practices is much higher costs of organic production, but is that true or will we sooner or later pay for our indiscriminate use of toxins? There is no doubt that eating organic products helps to strengthen our immune system, which means staying away from doctors and medications, not having to miss work and, eventually, reach old age without suffering. Therefore, throughout this book we encourage you to eat organic foods whenever possible. Also keep in mind that the energy content is much higher in organic products than in industrial products and therefore you will have to purchase a lesser amount.

WHY CHOOSE THEM

The Soil Association, an institution that supports and certifies organic products, proposes ten good reasons for preferring organic foods:

1. Protect future generations.
2. Pay the actual cost of authentic food.
3. Have guarantees that are not dependent on large corporations.
4. Protect water quality.
5. Enjoy foods that are high quality.
6. Avoid eating synthetic products.
7. Reduce global warming and save energy.
8. Prevent soil erosion.
9. Help small growers.
10. Help restore biodiversity.

Superfoods

vid news readers may feel a bit disappointed to note that superfoods have little to do with new technologies. What's more, quality depends precisely on traditional farming practices.

The thing that has changed since our grandmothers brewed teas to drink whenever they felt sick, is that now many home remedies have scientific backing. Science supports certain traditions and shed simple beliefs. Foods that are consumed in various Western regions since time immemorial, plus some from Eastern cultures are a natural treasure that both gratify the palate and have a wealth of natural therapeutic properties. Most superfoods belong to the plant kingdom because, according to experts, they are the best way to maintain optimal health or to recover it after an illness. However, this book is not geared only to readers who already know this information. Meat eaters should also opt for organic meat; otherwise they are taking risks with their food. You can find more information in various graphs and charts throughout this book.

"Only fresh, live foods will teach man the truth." (Pythagoras, c. 6th Century BC)

Food for hormonal problems

or many women with menstrual or menopausal problems, the term "estrogen" is already familiar, since it is the female sex hormone. Hormonal changes that women undergo throughout their lives may cause mild discomfort and severe pain, even migraines, a symptom that goes far beyond a headache. The pharmaceutical industry offers a wide range of drugs to relieve this monthly discomfort. However, there are foods that can help with these symptoms without any side effects. Hormonal problems are due to changes causing estrogen levels in the blood to rise and fall precipitously, and that's where certain foods can act to prevent estrogen levels from increasing as much.

Pain experienced during these hormonal changes is associated with a substance called "prostaglandin," of which there are several types. Some relieve inflammation and pain (PGE1 and PGE3) and the other PGE2 is related to inflammation, muscle contractions, compression of the blood vessels, and pain.

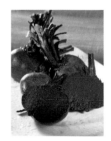

Foods that are to be avoided

• Food containing **harmful fats:** fries, snacks, conventional peanut butter, almost all pastries, and food preserved in oil.

Animal products (meat of any kind, eggs, cheese, milk, and other dairy products).

• **Industrial, plant-based, or animal fats** (butter, margarine, and cooking oils).

Before the start of the menstrual period, the glands produce large amounts of prostaglandins that are released during menstruation constricting blood vessels in the uterus, contracting muscles, causing painful cramps. In addition, upon entering the bloodstream prostaglandins can cause headaches, nausea, and diarrhea. Painkillers and anti-inflammatory drugs that are often prescribed to relieve pain reduce the production of prostaglandins. But is it possible to eliminate pain naturally? According to experiments conducted by Dr. Neal Barnard, an authority in the field of dietary therapy, some foods can trigger pain and other foods can make them disappear. With menstrual discomfort, prostaglandins form from fats remains stored in cell membranes.

After many tests done in women with severe cramps, it was found that a diet devoid of fat reduced estrogen levels significantly. And if that were not enough, researchers working on cancer have added merit to this phenomenon, because a decreased level of estrogen in the blood will help reduce the risk of breast cancer since there is not enough incentive for cancer cells to reproduce.

When periods are particularly painful, changes in diet can be very beneficial. Many women who replace animal products with vegetables and grains have noticed a big improvement. By eating a much smaller amount of fat, estrogen production decreases.

However, changes in eating habits must be made with certain precautions to prevent nutritional deficiencies. The following table indicates which foods to eat and which to avoid.

BREAST DISCOMFORT

Estrogen is also responsible for breast development during puberty. Sometimes, its concentration in the breasts may cause discomfort and pain. These dietary recommendations can also help in such cases. Moreover, some research points to coffee, tea, and chocolate as possible culprits for pain. Although results are not yet clear enough, try to drink them less often while menstruating.

Eat more...

• **Whole grains** (either as cereal or as flakes, bread, or drinks).
• **Fruits and vegetables** (all kinds and in large quantities).

• **Soy** (either sprouts, beans, tofu, or tempeh).

HELPFUL DIETARY SUPPLEMENTS

In addition to changing what we eat, the following list of supplements are highly recommended as part of a healthy diet.

• **ALA and GLA essential fatty acids.** In reference to prostaglandins, we already saw a bit about PGE1 (prostaglandin E1) and PGE3 (prostaglandin E3). They are available in health food stores in the form of tablets containing two types of vegetable fat: alpha-linolenic acid (ALA) and gamma-linolenic acid (GLA). The first type is directly responsible for the production of PGE3 and is found in vegetables, fruits, legumes, wheat germ, flax oil, and walnuts. It is an omega-3, which also includes fish oil. The second type is PGE1 and is present in borage oil, evening primrose oil, currant oil, hemp oil, and spirulina. Evening primrose oil and borage oil give great results and are available as capsules in pharmacies and specialty stores.

As we can see, it is not necessary to eliminate all types of fat from our diet. Just pay attention to which ones produce estrogen and which ones produce prostaglandins.

Most naturopaths do not recommend that you take them over long periods of time, but rather just before the menstrual period. Moreover, bear in mind that if pain is accompanied by physical and psychological disorders such as fluid retention, rashes, anxiety, binge eating, depression, irritability, mood swings, tension, or nerves, you should talk to your health care provider about combining supplements with more conventional treatments.

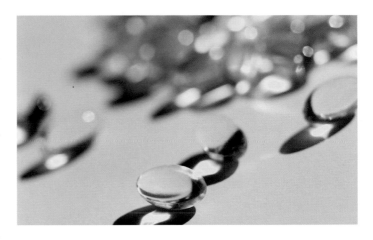

• **Calcium.** A balance of calcium may help reduce menstrual pain. There are different types of calcium supplements: calcium carbonate (highly recommended because it is absorbed more easily), calcium citrate, and calcium-magnesium. However, for better calcium absorption it is much more important to avoid foods that contribute to decalcification, such as animal protein, excess sugar, salt or alcohol, refined sugars, diuretics, and tobacco.

• **Soy isoflavones.** Phytoestrogens that help lower overall estrogenic activity.

• **Vitamin B6 or pyridoxine.** Apparently, this vitamin increases the production of neurotransmitters that eliminate the sensation of pain. It also helps expel estrogen from the liver. Very good results are obtained by combining it with magnesium or, even better, with GLA.

Evening primrose oil capsules provide very beneficial essential fatty acids to help alleviate hormonal problems.

Plants such as alfalfa or licorice have phytoestrogenic activity and can be taken as supplements

When should you take phytoestrogens?

- Whenever you are suffering from PMS.
- If you have hormonal irregularities.
- In case of infertility (without an exact health reason).

- During and after menopause. As the body produces less estrogen, phytoestrogens can help lessen typical symptoms of menopause.

Where can we find them?

- Vegetables: potatoes, yams, sweet potatoes, fennel, carrots, and beets.
- Legumes: soybeans (in all its forms), lentils (especially in germinated form), peas, beans (white, pinto, black, red), green beans, garbanzo (especially in germinated form).

- Grains: brown rice, oats, pearl barley, rye.
- Seeds: sesame, flax.
- Fruit: cherries, dates, apples, pomegranates.
- Aromatic herbs and other herbs: anise, sage, garlic, hops, truffles.

• **Yam.** It is a precursor to natural progesterone, a hormone that counteracts estrogen during ovulation. The supplement is a natural preparation whose active ingredient is identical to human progesterone. Research studies have shown that the amount present in cooked food is not enough, so progesterone is isolated in adequate quantities for it to have benefits. It is also possible to find topical cream containing yam to supplement estrogen in menopausal women. Ask your naturopath about using yams to balance your hormones.

• **Phytoestrogens.** Nature gives us "good" hormones: phytohormones or phytoestrogens. They are plant-derived estrogens that reduce the effects of estrogen. Some plants are richer in phytohormones than others.

It is believed that vegetarians have a higher level of phytoestrogens than people who follow a mixed diet because vegetarians tend to choose foods more carefully, preferring fresh and organic foods to take advantage of the synergy that occurs between plants, enhancing their benefits, when consumed in enough amounts, and because eating animal-based foods could negatively impact phytoestrogen levels in the body. So far this information is still unconfirmed, but it is certain that animal products are often the source of many ailments.

The proper diet

By remembering to eat fruits, vegetables, and whole grains and using the list of foods with the highest amount of phytoestrogens, you will be able to create your own menus, and make them healthy as well as tasty.

Food to prevent premature aging

There are two buzzwords in today's world of health foods: "free radicals" and "antioxidants" —just like in the movies, the "villains" and the "heroes." Antioxidants have always existed; free radicals are the novelty. But who are these "villains"? Free radicals are very unstable and destructive molecules (if they reproduce uncontrollably) that form when cells break up.

They have a toxic effect on the body's cells, alter its tissues, and cause premature or accelerated aging process known as "cellular oxidation" as well as cancer and other conditions. Free radicals have increased as modern life progresses: environmental pollution, toxic chemicals, "addiction" to medications, physical and emotional stress, tobacco, radiation exposure, inadequate food or GMOs, sunbathing . . .

All these factors create free radicals, whose harmful effects are reversed by the antioxidant "brigade," which are present in many foods as well as in dietary supplements (curiously enough there is an antioxidant complex called "Commando 2000"). But the benefits of antioxidants are not limited to combating premature aging or helping to prevent cancer; they are also useful as treatments for arthritis, chronic fatigue, and heart disorders.

CANCER PREVENTIVE ANTIOXIDANTS

"Cancer" is one of those dreaded things we wish we would never have to talk about much less suffer from. But before we talk about prevention, we have to tackle two questions: How does it start? And what causes it? The onset of cancer occurs when a cell starts to grow out of control and splits again and again, becoming a mass invading tissue, in some specific body part.

Risk for cancer is due to our genetic makeup or to other factors such as diet or pollution (tobacco, radiation, toxic chemicals). There are studies confirming that thirty to sixty percent of cancer cases are caused by eating certain foods that stimulate the production of cancer cells.

Risk for cancer can stem from our genetic makeup or other factors such as diet or pollution.

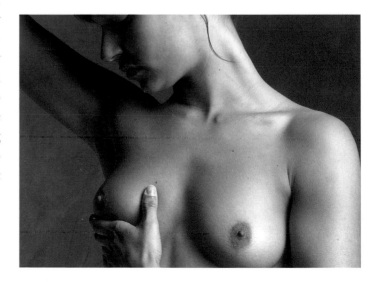

Diets rich in vegetables, fruits, and whole grains reduce the risk of cancer.

But this should not be an alarming statistic because you need to take into account other factors and especially our best weapon: a strengthened immune system. What we eat is so important that the World Cancer Research Fund and American Institute for Cancer Research has concluded that proper nutrition can reduce incidences of several types of cancer by up to forty percent. Cancers that are more closely related to diet appear in organs that are controlled by sex hormones (prostate, breast, uterus, and ovaries) and also in gastrointestinal organs (stomach, esophagus, liver, pancreas, and colon). Research studies comparing different societies like Japanese versus US have identified two predominant constants: diets rich in animal products and high in fat tend to increase cancer risk, while vegetables, fruits, grains, and legumes tend to lower the risk. In addition, it is suspected that certain foodspromote the development of various cancers.

• **Breast cancer.** It is closely related to estrogen production. It is recommended that we eliminate fats, especially animal fats, and increase our fiber intake through grains and vegetables. Watch out with dairy! The Association of Physicians for Responsible Medicine, in Washington, discovered that the problem was not only with milk fat but also with the estrogen it contains. Indeed, cattle are kept in continuous state of nursing for maximum milk productivity, but more importantly, milk contains growth factors to help calves grow quickly. One, called IGF-1, stimulates the development of cancer cells more than estrogen itself.

In addition, alcohol may also lead to breast cancer: one drink a day can increase the risk factor by more than fifty percent.

• **Cancer of the uterus and ovaries.** Studies at Johns Hopkins revealed that the higher the cholesterol, the higher the risk for ovarian cancer. Animal fats represent again the role of "bad guys" because they are not only responsible for elevating cholesterol levels, but they are also linked to the production of estrogen, hormones closely linked with the sexual organs.

Harvard University also found another reason for us to avoid dairy products: galactose, a sugar potentially dangerous to the ovaries. Skimmed products are also included in this group.

• **Prostate cancer.** Just as women have problems with the production of estrogen, men have problems with a hormone called testosterone. Fat intake stimulates the production of testosterone which in turn stimulates the development of cancer cells.

• **Cancer of the digestive system.** Esophageal cancer is usually associated with frequently drinking hot beverages, eating canned food, or drinking alcohol and smoking, which greatly increases risk for cancer.

Stomach cancer is linked to smoked and salted foods.

Pancreatic cancer is thought to be influenced by eating meat and drinking alcohol and coffee.

Colon cancer (very closely linked to everything we eat, because everything ends up there), is caused by eating meat, particularly beef and chicken. Problems arise precisely when we cook meat before eating it. When we heat up animal proteins, they produce a carcinogenic substance called "heterocyclic amines."

These data are not just theories; they tend to appear again and again in cancer statistics. Fortunately, there are many substances with anti-cancer properties in certain antioxidants.

ANTIOXIDANTS TO PREVENT PREMATURE AGING

Old age is a natural and inevitable process that we all go through at some point. Oftentimes we think of this period of life as one with impairment or disease, but could things be different?

Outside of expensive procedures such as cosmetic surgery, implants, or rejuvenating treatments with young cells, there are other more accessible methods for becoming healthy and beautiful seniors: some exercise, a sense of humor, taking it slow, meditating, and of course, following a healthy diet. Many young people believe they are immune to toxins so they eat a lot of fast food, fried snacks, animal fats, carbonated soft drinks, sugar and dyes, or they are surrounded in a thick cloud of tobacco. "Why not?" they ask. "At the end of the day nobody dies from eating hotdogs

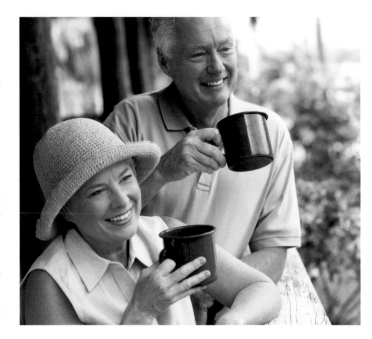

with bacon and fries, drinking a cola, and having a coffee while smoking a cigarette."

Early on, the body begins to send small warnings: heartburn, headache, occasionally vomiting . . . If these bad habits continue, the body will eventually accumulate toxins and suffer many types of diseases. The fewer bad habits we have, the more we will enjoy better health.

There are a variety of foods that can help us enjoy a healthy old age.

Old age is a natural and inevitable process that does not have to be associated with deterioration and disease.

At this point, we should mention superfoods with antioxidant properties that can defend against cell damage.

NATURAL ANTIOXIDANTS

• **Algae.** This amazing seaweed provides us with a good amount of vitamin E, provitamin A (beta carotene), and linoleic and alpha-linolenic acids. This particular synergy of substances contained in algae acts against premature aging and protects the skin and mucous membranes from free radicals.

• **Garlic and onion.** Research shows that both have "organosulfur" compounds that stimulate the production of enzymes that neutralize carcinogens. Maximum benefits are obtained from eating them raw, although red onion slightly retains more of its properties when exposed to moderate heat due to the presence of an antioxidant substance called "quercetin."

Garlic also contains selenium and germanium (provided that the soil in which it was cultivated also contains these minerals), which protect the body against aging due to free radicals, and help to eliminate heavy metals like mercury and lead. It also provides defenses against radiation and cancer.

• **Blueberries.** They have an extraordinary amount of antioxidants and a great ability to neutralize free radicals and destroy molecules that can damage DNA. Its secret lies in its blue pigments that contain anthocyanins, which destroy some of the most common carcinogens. Anthocyanins are also found in other fruits such as plums, cherries, and currants.

• **Carotenes.** They are not foods themselves, but rather antioxidants that are found in yellow or orange vegetables (carrots, sweet potatoes, squash, peach, or apricot) or leafy greens such as spinach and parsley.

Just a hundredth of a milligram of carotene in the liver works as a major reserve of vitamin A for growth and rejuvenation.

Carotenes are able to eliminate free radicals, even better than vitamin E. Although most research has focused on beta-carotene, there are hundreds of antioxidant carotenoids (alpha carotene, gamma carotene, lycopene . . .).

The benefits of carrots

Since 1922 studies have shown that vitamin A prevents cancerous degeneration in epithelial cells. Starting in 1981 a great number of studies have been conducted on how vitamins may protect against cancer. The British Association for Cancer Research has published findings that make a direct connection between the risk of cancer and the amount of beta-carotene we eat.

Carrots, which are rich in beta carotene, are a precursor of provitamin A, which is converted to vitamin A once it is synthesized in the liver. As if that were not enough, eating carrots improves our eyesight and beautifies our skin.

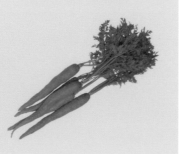

- **Citrus.** We particularly refer to oranges, lemons, and limes containing an abundant amount of limonene. Limonene is a substance that stimulates the natural production of a class of enzymes that prepare killer cells, that is, they destroy cancer cells. Citrus fruits also contain glucarase, a component that deactivates carcinogens and expels them from the body. On the other hand, we cannot forget one of the most recognized antioxidant vitamins: vitamin C, which humans cannot synthesize, so we need an external daily intake. Note that men's daily needs are around 75 to 100 mg, and from 70 to 100 mg for women, but during pregnancy and lactation a higher dose is required. Half a cup (100 ml) of juice contains about 50 mg of vitamin C. Start each day by drinking the juice of one lemon mixed with some water to prevent premature aging.

- **Cruciferae.** This family, consisting of white cabbage, red cabbage, Brussels sprouts, cauliflower, and broccoli are excellent antioxidants. The anticancer properties of broccoli were some of the first to be demonstrated and they continue to place it among the most powerful. As we saw in the chapter on nutraceuticals, its active ingredient is sulforaphane, a substance that stimulates the body to produce an enzyme that deactivates carcinogens. They also have a lot of vitamin C. Eating crucifers often helps us stay healthy in old age.

- **Miso.** This is a paste obtained by fermenting yellow soy beans, so it contains live lactobacteria that is very beneficial for our bodies. The Japanese attribute their good health and longevity to miso, which is why they are never without miso at the table.

This soy derivative contains a substance called "citicoline" that attracts, absorbs, and eliminates radioactivity from the human body. Another component is the miraculous melanoidin, which inhibits free radicals. Surely that's one good reason why Japanese traffic cops eat it so much, as for much of the day they are exposed to high levels of pollution.

- **Cayenne pepper.** It has a good amount of capsaicin, a powerful antioxidant that prevents the fatal mix of nitrites and amines, and almost completely neutralizes the resulting carcinogens. It can also prevent carcinogens in tobacco smoke from adhering to DNA, which prevents, for example, the development of lung cancer. But it is always best to quit smoking and not eat chilies continuously.

- **Beet.** In a German study conducted in 1994 with over sixty varieties of fruits and vegetables, it was shown that the beet contains several of the most potent anticancer agents.

Sauerkraut is a German dish often used as a garnish for various dishes. Its antioxidant and anticancer qualities make it one of the most recommended foods for a healthy diet.

Fermented foods

Known for having a high nutritional value, sprouts are considered "fountains of youth" for their optimal combination of antioxidants and enzymes. Green lentil sprouts are among the most desirable since they contain substances that slow down the aging process.

How the grain germinates

Using a compartmentalized germinator

· First day:

Place seeds in a container, pour a glass of water, and cover.

· Second day:

Place some seeds into another container then pour over the seeds from the previous day, add another glass of water, and cover.

· Third day:

Repeat this process with new seeds and another container.

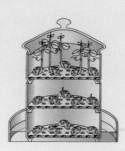

Using a jar

· First day:

Place seeds in a jar, cover them with water, cover the jar with gauze and secure it with a rubber band. Within an hour, turn it over and drain out excess water.

· Second day:

Shake the jar, flip it over on to a plate and tilt it slightly so that the seeds are not immersed in the decanted water. You can repeat the same step as the previous day using another jar.

· Third day:

Shake both jars just as you did the previous day and prepare a new jar with seeds.

Using a strainer

· First day:

Fill a large strainer with seeds. Then for one hour, immerse it in a container filled with water.

· Second day:

Rinse the seeds and place the strainer in a bowl. At the end of the day, rinse the seeds again.

· Third day:

Rinse the seeds in the morning and in the evening.

Using any of these three methods, the seeds can be eaten after the third or fourth day.

One of them, the betacyanin, is what gives it its characteristic color. Fresh beets, not canned beets, have a lot of folic acid, which protects the body against heart disease and colon cancer.

• **Soy.** Soy is a plant rich in genistein, a substance with anti-cancer properties. Estrogens stimulate the growth of cancer cells in ovaries and breasts, but genistein acts to interrupt that process. Another quality is its vitamin E, an antioxidant that helps our skin.

• **Green Tea.** It is widely recognized in the East (and increasingly in the West) as a powerful antioxidant due to substances called "polyphenols." Once malignant cells are formed, one particular type of polyphenol, known as "epigallocatechin gallate" (EGCG), stops the spread of cancer and may even remove it without affecting healthy cells. For its ability to neutralize free radicals, green tea is one of the best preventive foods against premature aging.

• **Tomato.** Edward Giovanucci, epidemiologist from Harvard University, compared seventy-two experiments that examined the incidence of cancer among individuals according to the amount of tomato included in their diet, and found that the number of regular tomato eaters had 45% less incidence of cancer. Blood tests showed a high level of lycopene, an antioxidant that gives tomatoes their red coloring. Furthermore, it is believed that for lycopene to be released and for the body to absorb it, tomatoes should be cooked. For those with a tomato allergy, lycopene can be obtained from pink grapefruit, watermelon, and guava.

• **Red grape.** Much like blueberries, grapes contain anthocyanins and flavonoids that increase the power of vitamin C. US scientific studies have determined that grapes contain a substance called "resveratrol" that can prevent some types cancer. You can enjoy it as a refreshing juice (well-sealed and organic) to help eliminate toxins.

• **Peppers, raspberries, kiwi, strawberries.** They provide a lot of vitamin C.

HELPFUL DIETARY SUPPLEMENTS
Today, health food stores offer a wide range of antioxidants on the shelves: vitamins and minerals alone or in combination, in capsule or powder, juices, liquid capsules, tablets, etc. Before buying anything, talk to your doctor or naturopath about the best options for you. Below you will find a short description of antioxidants against aging and cell degeneration.

• **Green tea extract.** For those who do not have time to drink a couple of cups a day.

• **Germanium.** Essential against cancer and for boosting your immune system.

• **Wheat germ.** Contains various antioxidants, but it mostly has vitamin E, one of the best treatments for the skin. It can also reduce certain types of cancer. Sprinkle it in soups, or mix it with salads or muesli. Eat it as fresh as possible, make sure that it is organic, and keep it in the refrigerator because it goes rancid quickly. Another option is to get wheat germ oil that comes in gel capsules to prevent oxidation.

• **Selenium.** Nutrient that protects against pollution, and therefore against free radicals. In small doses, it can reduce the risk of prostate and colon cancer. Consult your physician to discuss your family history with cancer and ask about taking selenium supplements. Beware of self-medication: more than 1 mg per day can cause hair loss, fatigue, nausea, and vomiting.

Food and dietary supplements can help us boost our immune system and improve our health.

Three special anti-aging supplements

One of our common fears regarding old age, is that we will lose suppleness in our skin along with our memory. We will not delve into the complications of the human brain, but we can explore certain trending supplements that aid and protect our brain activity.

Phosphatidylserine

It is a phospholipid (phosphorus fat) that occurs naturally and though present throughout the body, it is especially concentrated in the brain. Its essential function is to protect brain function: for example, it helps with lack of concentration, improves memory, and increases overall brain performance.

Coenzyme Q_{10}

Also known as "ubiquinone," it is a substance found in body cells. It is good for many of the conditions mentioned in this book, but it can also help strengthen memory, increase energy, and it has antioxidant properties recommended for healthy aging.

Ginkgo biloba

It is a long-living tree revered by Chinese and Japanese cultures where it is considered an extraordinary remedy. In the West, tests concluded that it is extremely useful for old age disorders such as lack of concentration or memory, depression, or fatigue. It has even been used to treat Alzheimer's disease

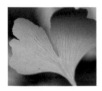

Ginkgo Biloba

• **Vitamins C and E.** These are two antioxidant vitamins that complement each other because they each fulfill many different functions in the body, so one does not replace the other. Vitamin E is fat soluble (dissolves in fat) and C is water-soluble (dissolves in water). Vitamin C supplements with bioflavonoids are the best because they act synergistically.

• **Vitamin A and beta carotene.** Protects mucous membranes against smog and cancer.

• **Antioxidant enzymes.** These are not digestive enzymes, but cellular enzymes in foods that need to be eaten raw to maximize their benefits, such as fruits, vegetables, sprouts, and wheatgrass. The main protective enzymes against free radicals are superoxide dismutase (SOD), glutathione peroxidase (GP), and catalase.

These enzymes quickly control free radicals in the body, three to ten times faster than antioxidant nutrients. These enzymes locate, neutralize, and recycle certain substances that are harmful to the body. For example, catalase "disarms" hydrogen peroxide (responsible for cell damage from free radicals) and converts it into oxygen and water. The most important synergy occurs between superoxide dismutase and catalase. It is available in food stores in tablet form, although some complex antioxidants may be even more effective.

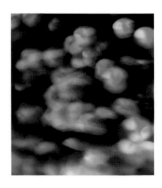

Food to strengthen the joints

Joint conditions (arthritis, osteoarthritis, chronic rheumatism, gout, etc.) are closely linked to toxic and waste substances that accumulate around the joints and cause inflammation and pain.

These are very intense pains due to muscle contraction caused by local tissue asphyxia, in which circulation slows and decreases considerably. The result is an insufficient blood flow and tissues that lack oxygen; that is why massaging the affected area is useful by activating circulation and channeling out waste. In addition to the accumulated toxins and free radicals in various forms, there are a number of foods that trigger pain while other foods help prevent them. Although there is a lot of controversy about how food is involved in joint pain, it does not hurt to try to make some improvements in your diet. If it means mitigating or eliminating pain, why not try? Before covering the topic of food, we will learn about some of the most common joint diseases.

• **Arthritis.** Painful inflammation of tissues surrounding the joints. Lesions first reach the cartilage (covering surface of the bones), then the bones, and then perhaps result in deformation or motor impairment. Unlike osteoarthritis, arthritis is not related to age and even the young can suffer from it. The question is: Is there any chance of stopping the damage, of mitigating the pain? It is believed that free radicals, those unstable and destructive molecules (when they grow uncontrollably) have a toxic effect on cells, they cause pain, and they are a real problem for inflamed joints. In fact, we could say that they are toxins that attack the joints (among other things). The antidote to neutralizing them is antioxidants, substances that are naturally present in many minerals and vegetables.

• **Arthrosis.** Chronic degenerative disease that can cause joint deformity that usually appears after the age forty. Over the years, cartilage that lines the contact surface of bones "shrinks," losing thickness and may virtually disappear in the most serious cases. One of the most frequently affected areas are the cervical vertebrae, where it causes difficulty to move the head easily and the most severe cases result in osteoarthritis of the hips that impedes walking.

• **Osteoarthritis.** It is also a degenerative joint disease that is a consequence of aging. One of the first things to do in cases of osteoarthritis is eliminate excess weight.

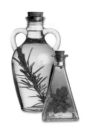

Excess iron and oils in the diet can accelerate damage produced by free radicals.

Vitamin E relieves pain and improves mobility in people with osteoarthritis.

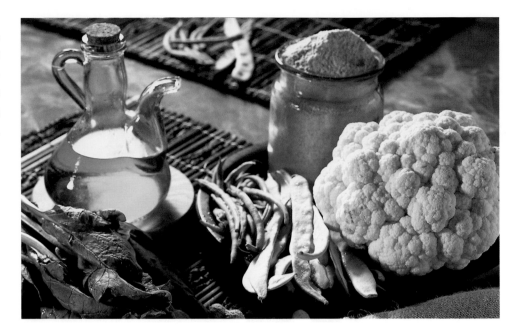

But why? Because every ten pounds (four and a half kilos) of excess weight increases the risk of osteoarthritis in the knees by thirty percent. Also, another issue that has been detected is that although this disease occurs after age sixty-five in both genders, women who have suffered from excess estrogen suffer more osteoarthritis than men. In the chapter about hormonal problems, we learned that estrogen is produced by fat cells, so if you need to start losing weight, nothing beats eliminating estrogen production by avoiding fatty foods and increasing the amount of fruits, vegetables, whole grains, and legumes you eat.

Not all people with arthritis have trouble with the same food. It varies from one person to another, but some foods are "frequent culprits."

• **Rheumatoid arthritis.**

It is one of the most serious joint problems as it brings on pain, bleeding, and joint deformities over time. This disease (which is more common in women over fifty) does not occur as a result of old age; instead it is an "autoimmune" illness because the body attacks itself. White blood cells whose job is to defend against bacteria, viruses, and cancer cells, instead begin attacking tissues lining the joints. Some foods trigger this reaction. Although it may sound strange, just as some foods cause a series of reactions for allergy sufferers, in the case of arthritis there are also foods that can cause a painful reaction for people with intolerance. To determine whether food is related to arthritis, a group of medical researchers subjected patients to a controlled fasting period for several days, after which most patients felt relief from pain and remarkable improvement.

Then as the study went along, a system of food elimination was used in order to identify which ones caused more problems. Moreover, not all people have food intolerances, but those who do have them and know which foods make them feel bad, are able to enjoy a much better diet.

• **Gout.** Symptoms that signal gout resemble those that affect the liver: coated tongue, vomiting, eructation, hemorrhoids, constipation alternating with diarrhea, blood in the urine, and depression. Sudden attacks begin with sharp pain that starts in the big toe and then spreads to other joints.

The joints are filled with uric acid crystals. Unlike many animal species that have enzymes that rapidly eliminate uric acid from the body, humans retain it; perhaps because it is a powerful antioxidant like vitamin C. Some people retain uric acid in the joints where white blood cells try to "crush" it, causing inflammation and pain. Gout differs from other rheumatic attacks mainly because veins will dilate, possibly due to excess waste in the blood, and if it is not monitored early on, it can lead to other disorders (nephritis, hypertension, urea). The worst triggers for gout attacks are eating meat and drinking alcohol, especially anchovies, shellfish, sardines, organ meats, and beer.

People with gout are more likely to have a seizure during dietary changes. It is best to keep taking medication (if you already do so) during the transition into better eating habits (eliminating trigger foods and eating more fruits, vegetables, whole grains, and legumes) and consult with your doctor

Soothing compress for gout

Take a fresh cabbage leaf, crush it with a rolling pin, apply it to the affected area, and leave it there until there is relief.

about possibly continuing or stopping your medications.

• **Rheumatoid arthritis of the cervical spine.** There are many types of rheumatism affecting the cervical spine. Two are particularly serious: spondylitis and rheumatism which deforms the spine. The first is caused by acute demineralization with intermittent pain that usually occurs at night. After the attack, the consequences are loss of flexibility of the spine and difficulty in movement. Rheumatism deforms the vertebrae by compressing and wearing down cartilage. The lumbar vertebrae and the neck are usually the most affected.

There is a very unique folk remedy for joint pain: a bee sting. Apparently the poison of these insects is not as bad as you think, since it could have a substance that reduces inflammation in the joints. However, allergy sufferers can be severely affected by this remedy.

GETTING TO THE ROOT OF THE PROBLEM

Fasting is a good way to find out if any of the foods that you eat are causing problems. It is very good for the body, as it allows you to get rid of toxins, which is an important part of getting healthy. There is no need to associate fasting with suffering. If you follow certain recommendations, you will not go hungry and you will have more energy, and your blood and organs will feel clean.

Fasting

Fasting is a therapeutic method that is controversial among doctors because of the mistrust for any therapeutic method that costs nothing. Although it has nothing to do with anorexia, some have come to associate it with this disorder.

The decision to stop eating for a while does not have to do with wanting to lose weight: therapeutic fasting helps eliminate toxins and cleanse the body of substances generated by heavy foods or eating poorly, which can eventually cause diseases.

The simplest fasting lasts between 24 and 72 hours.

Extending it longer without the supervision of a doctor can be dangerous.

Before fasting, take into account your health and age. Children, adolescents, and those who feel physical or mental weakness should abstain from fasting.

Types of fasting
1) **Completely avoid ingesting solid foods.** Only drink mineral water in large quantities.
2) Replace solid food with **fruit juices**.
3) Replace solid foods with **water, soups, and fruit juices**.
4) **Sap and lemon juice treatment**.

Although foods pose no problem for most people, there are patients with an intolerance to certain foods, like chocolate, malt, alcoholic drinks, bananas, soy products, products with nitrites, onion, cane sugar, and various spices, such as coriander, mint, and cardamom.

Whether other foods cause more or less serious disorders is still unknown. Obviously, there are others that may be equally or more harmful, although usually only in isolated cases. If you suspect that a certain food item is causing you problems, follow an elimination diet.

DIET PLAN

People suffering from joint pain quickly turn to drugs to curb inflammation, pain, and despair that comes with it. Sometimes drugs are a great relief, but other times they are not as effective as expected and they fail to solve the problem, often causing side effects.

One way to reduce discomfort is to test out a new diet: for a month, you will have to avoid any food that may cause discomfort. It is very likely that after this time you will notice some improvement, although chronic inflammation in the joints can take longer to improve.

From there on, it is ideal to continue avoiding foods that are associated with joint pain and prepare different menus with foods that do not cause inflammation or pain.

Thanks to various medical and nutritional studies, we know that a wide range of products that we usually eat may cause certain disorders.

In various trials, patients were urged to reintroduce foods that had previously been eliminated from their diet to determine which foods were most problematic. Doing this may cause worsening in the patient but it allows you to treat the problem more effectively. To avoid a strong relapse, you can bring back one food at a time. It is advisable to let a couple of weeks go by before examining another food item. If eliminating certain foods from the list does not help, may be the problem is in other foods. To identify them, do as follows: first eat only safe foods; once joint pain is relieved, add good quantities of food that you eat regularly (not shown in any of the two lists) to see which one is the most problematic. Sometimes all it takes is a small amount for inflammation and pain to appear. Other times, a greater amount is needed. The important thing is to discover what it is. Sometimes it is one of our favorite foods so we'll have to get used to not having it.

Another option to determine our food intolerance is undergoing special analysis to discover the worst enemies of our joints, but it is a rather expensive method.

Finally, after discovering the main enemies of your joints, keep eating raw fruits and vegetables. In fact, start to eat them even more often.

HELPFUL DIETARY SUPPLEMENTS

• **ALA and GLA fatty acids.** In the chapter on food for hormonal problems, we saw how substances called "prostaglandins" have much to do with pain and inflammation. Two prostaglandins can be obtained through natural fats and have an anti-inflammatory action on the joints without side effects: prostaglandin E1 and E3. Most importantly, however, is knowing what and where those natural fats are. They are essential fatty acids because we need to obtain them in adequate levels through food. One is alpha-linolenic acid (ALA, it is easier to remember it as an acronym), which is an omega-3 fatty acid and is present in some fruits and vegetables and, in a much more concentrated way, in flaxseed oil (which has the highest ALA content), walnut oil, and wheat germ.

Foods that can cause disorders

Oats	Citrus	Wheat
Coffee	Eggs	Nuts
Meat (any animal meat and meat products)	Corn	Dairy (any animal-derived milk and dairy products: cheese, yogurt, cottage cheese, etc.)
	Seafood	
Rye (including flours, flakes, and drinks)	Potatoes	
	Tomatoes	

Foods that do not cause pain or inflammation

Mineral water	Maple syrup	beets, asparagus,
Brown rice	Sea salt in small amounts	spinach, lettuce, green
Cooked or dried fruits (cranberries, prunes, raisins, cherries, pears)	Cooked vegetables (artichokes, broccoli,	beans, squash, sweet potato, tapioca).

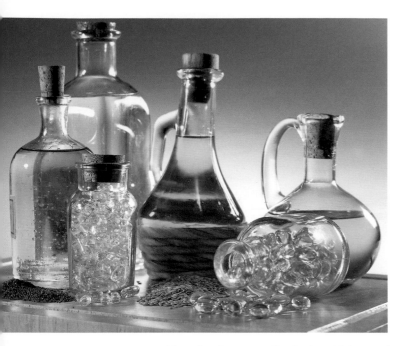

Fatty acids in flaxseed oil and borage oil have anti-inflammatory action on joints.

plus vitamin E, which protects oils from oxidation. You can find these oil blends in capsules. However, before you start taking any of these, talk to your doctor who will indicate the most appropriate dose for you. EPA (eicosapentaenoic acid) is an omega-3 fatty acid from fish oils from cold seas; it helps rheumatoid arthritis by inhibiting inflammation.

• **Antioxidants.** Finally, do not forget antioxidant supplements that act as defenses against free radicals in the joints. In particular, vitamin E relieves pain and improves mobility in people with osteoarthritis. Moreover, spirulina also contains vitamin E and carotene.

The other is gamma-linolenic acid (or GLA), which is an omega-6 found only in borage oil (containing the highest proportion of GLA), evening primrose oil, blackcurrant oil, hemp oil, and spirulina. Animal fats and cooking oils negatively affect hormonal functions, by increasing estrogen levels, but they are also harmful because they result in inflammation. So, a diet that includes animal products (meat), dairy products, and oily foods can result in an accumulation of harmful fat that causes inflammation. On the other hand, ALA and GLA fatty acids may help you see positive changes.

As a treatment for arthritis, take supplements that contain more GLA and ALA, flaxseed oil, and borage oil (or evening primrose oil)

MORE NATURAL ANTI-INFLAMMATORIES
In addition to ALA and GLA, there are additional natural products that act against pain or inflammation.

• **Spirulina.** It is a blue freshwater algae that comes from the tropics. Due to its concentration of antioxidants and GLA fatty acids, it protects against free radicals and it also has anti-inflammatory action.

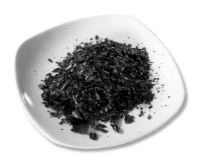

Warning
GLA is not recommended for pregnant women because as a hormonal regulator, it can cause a miscarriage.

- **Ginger.** This ancient root has been used for centuries in Indian Ayurvedic medicine as a treatment for arthritis. It is very beneficial to the body, especially because it has an effective anti-inflammatory action. Simply take one teaspoon or half a teaspoon of ginger powder every day. If you are using fresh ginger, then use more.

- **Black currant.** The leaves and buds of the plant are recognized as antirheumatic due to flavonoids which stimulate the secretion of anti-inflammatory substances. It has been dubbed "natural cortisone" though without its many drawbacks. Its fruit juice is also recommended as an anti-inflammatory treatment. You can also brew it (30 to 150 currants for every 4 cups (10 to 50 g per liter) of water) or drink it as an extract.

- **Noni.** This is the *Morinda citrifolia* plant that is native to the South Pacific islands. It is one of the newest additions to the world of nutraceutical supplements in the West, but it has been used for medicinal purposes for thousands of years by the native people of Hawaii and Polynesia. According to research on the properties of the fruit of this tree, its regenerative power is associated with xeronine, an alkaloid that works at the cellular level and strengthens the immune system. It has notable effects in cases of joint pain and rheumatism, and relieves symptoms of arthritis, osteoarthritis, rheumatoid arthritis, and gout.

- **Cayenne pepper.** Its strength is due to its capsaicin, an ingredient that gives it its spiciness. But you do not have to eat it with spaghetti because there are cayenne pepper capsules.

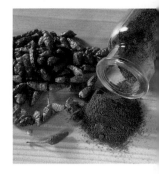

Cayenne pepper or chilies.

Food for healthy bones

O steoporosis is a disease that accompanies menopause, but it is not an exclusively female disorder since many men also suffer from it. Osteoporosis ("porous bones") is characterized by the gradual loss of bone density: pores get larger and bones become weaker, resulting in fractures. Later in life, even a small blow can cause a fragile bone to break. This problem is not always due to a lack of calcium in the diet. Some foods absorb calcium that should be going into the bones, causing a calcium deficiency. But there are other factors such as sedentary lifestyle, a strong genetic predisposition, digestive difficulty absorbing calcium, and lack of other nutrients such as certain vitamins and minerals, especially magnesium. And what about women who are going through menopause? Now we'll see how that phase relates to osteoporosis and the importance of progesterone.

PROGESTERONE

Menopause stops ovulation which ceases production of progesterone, the hormone that stimulates the production of osteoblasts (bone cells responsible for bone formation). This means that a lack of progesterone implies insufficient osteoblast activity and, therefore, reduced production of new bone. This explains why osteoporosis affects women starting at about age forty-five, at the onset of menopause.

But the good news is that we can naturally replenish a damaged bone with a new, healthy bone. This is possible using natural progesterone, an exact copy of human progesterone that is especially found in yams and soybeans.

You can also find isolated natural progesterone in the form of an ointment that is applied on the skin and then absorbed into the bloodstream. There it reaches the "damaged" bone and "summons" osteoblasts to build new bone. Apparently, natural progesterone can cause bone density to increase at a sufficient rate to heal fractures.

ABSORBING THE MOST AMOUNT OF CALCIUM

Although bones need calcium that does not mean you should have milk, cheese, or custard at all times, because although these foods contain plenty of calcium, the body does not easily absorb it. This is because over time we lose the enzyme that digests lactose.

Moreover, dairy that is not organic may have an amount of toxic waste or additives that should be avoided. Also, some people are lactose intolerant. Statistics show that countries with the highest consumption of dairy products are those with the highest incidence of osteoporosis, and the reason is that their diet is rich in fat and meat, two substances involved in calcium metabolism.

There are other foods, such as some seeds and vegetables, whose content of absorbable calcium is much higher.

In addition to calcium, take vitamin D and magnesium, two nutrients that help you absorb calcium better. Vitamin D is synthesized by sunlight (fifteen minutes, three times per week is all you need), but it can also be obtained from certain dietary supplements. Magnesium is found in many foods, especially brown rice and dark legumes.

DECALCIFICATION

To maintain good bone health, it is important to consider foods that provide calcium as well as those that absorb it.

Kefir

Kefir is an exception within dairy, since it is fermented milk, it is rich in bacteria and yeast, and it has great benefits for the body. These bacteria ferment milk through an alcoholic reaction that breaks down nutrients, which allows lactose intolerant people to drink it and prevent osteoporosis.

• **Animal proteins.** Eating a diet in which red meat, poultry, fish, and eggs are predominant tends to cause metabolic acidosis, a disorder that the body aims to eliminate quickly using calcium from the bones.

• **Diuretics and laxatives.** Promote mineral loss.

• **Sodium.** Increases urinary calcium excretion. To prevent this loss, avoid eating salty foods or canned products that have a large proportion of sodium components. It is also important to limit salt in cooking and at the table. It has been shown that reducing sodium intake to 1 to 2 grams per day can save you an average of 160 mg of calcium daily.

• **Tobacco.** Smokers lose calcium on top of their wellbeing and their money. Smoking has been found to increase the risk of osteoporosis in women. Tobacco is well known for the many problems it causes, for creating addiction, and for how difficult it can be for some people to quit.

• **Lack of exercise.** Daily exercise is one of the best ways to stay in good health. If done outdoors, oxygen will be of better quality and sunlight will tone your skin and ensure the formation of vitamin D.

• **Sugary sodas.** Cola in particular has a high phosphorus content (in the form of phosphoric acid) and while this mineral is useful in small amounts for calcium absorption, when it is in large quantities it has the opposite effect. Moreover, these drinks promote

Plant-derived foods with the most calcium

Poppyseed	1,450 mg/100 g
Iziki algae	1,400 mg/100 g
Wakame seaweed	1,380 mg/100 g
Arame seaweed	1,170 mg/100 g
Sesame seeds	783 mg/100 g
Hazelnuts	290 mg/100 g
Soybeans	260 mg/100 g
Almonds	240 mg/100 g
Chinese cabbage (also known as kale)	250 mg/100 g
Dried figs (about ten medium sized)	269 mg
Tofu	(1/2 cup) 258 mg
Watercress	180 mg/100 g
White beans (one cup, cooked)	161 mg

(An 8 ounce (200 ml) glass of milk has 240 mg calcium and 4 oz (125 g) of yogurt has 136 mg.)

acidosis, a disorder that our body must neutralize by using calcium from bones.

Moreover, avoid drinking excessive amounts of coffee, sugar, and alcohol, and eating refined (which are not whole grains: white bread, white rice, white flour) products as much as possible because they eliminate minerals from the body.

CALCIUM AT AN EARLY AGE
You do not have to be old to worry about your bone health.

Sesame seeds are small and hard, so because they cannot be chewed well we eliminate them without absorbing them. Therefore, to maximize their nutrients, grind them first or if you prefer, use gomasio, which is a condiment made with sesame.

How much calcium do we need?

The recommended daily dose is as follows:
• 800 mg for children aged 4 to 8 years.
• 1,300 mg until age 18.
• 1,000 mg until age 50.

• 1,200 mg for people over 50.
• 1,000 mg to prevent osteoporosis, starting at age 25.
• 1,500 mg for postmenopausal women.

It seems that "Western taste" of many children and adolescents includes many items that steal calcium and which over time can cause bone problems. A study involving adolescents who were given sugar and caffeine (found in conventional soft drinks) showed that caffeine tripled calcium loss in the three hours right after drinking it, and that sugar doubled the rate of calcium elimination through urine. That is, if children and adolescents drink milk and eat yogurt, whatever calcium they are able to absorb is lost due to the soft drinks they ingest.

The higher the bone mass is when they are done growing, the lower the risk of osteoporosis in old age.

OSTEOPOROSIS IN MEN

It occurs less often than in women. The most common causes include: significant amount of alcoholic drinks, testosterone in lower than normal amounts, decalcification through food, and insufficient levels of vitamin D.

Prevent it by eating few animal proteins, avoiding coffee, salt, alcohol, and tobacco as well as doing physical activity, and taking vitamin D supplements (or sun).

Food for a healthy heart

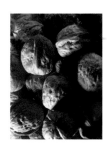

According to the experts, heart problems are closely linked to bad habits such as a diet rich in animal fats (saturated), smoking, lack of exercise, and stress. As we can see, almost all disorders are due to the same causes. Fortunately, there is always room for improvement.

The heart only begins to pose problems when blood vessels surrounding it (coronary arteries) accumulate residues left behind by "dirty" blood. From that moment on we will hear about good cholesterol, bad cholesterol, triglycerides, good fats, bad fats, HDL or LDL that indicate that our health is suffering.

Every discovery known about the effects of food on heart conditions is available to us. Even large corporations advertise the sale of new products not only without cholesterol, but also with added "good fats" that help combat it.

IS CHOLESTEROL THE SAME AS FAT?

A certain amount of cholesterol in the body is considered normal, but as with free radicals, problems begin when that number increases.

Helpful dietary supplements

• **Soy isoflavones**
Effective for preventing osteoporosis. As a precursor of progesterone, it can regenerate new bone that was previously damaged.

• **Silica**
Silica is a mineral that can be found in tablets, powder, or extract and it has been proven effective in combating diseases such as arthritis, rheumatism, and for strengthening bones.

• **Calcium**
Calcium carbonate or calcium citrate are both absorbed more easily and can be good sources.

• **Magnesium**
If the average calcium intake is set at 1,000 mg daily, its ideal complement is 500 mg of magnesium.

• **Vitamin D**
The sun can give it to you, but you can also find it in capsules.

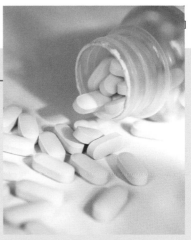

• A number of other vitamins and minerals are important, such as **vitamins A, B, C, E, K and minerals like boron, silicon, and zinc.**

Eating products that derive from animals is partly to blame. Like us, animals have an amount of stored cholesterol and when we eat meat, we add their cholesterol to our own body. In this case, the extra cholesterol particles in the blood are enough to gradually form plaques in the arteries, obstructing blood flow. Diets consisting of meat and animal products (eggs, butter, whole milk) are rich in cholesterol. For example, a 7 oz (200 g) fillet of beef contains approximately .006 oz (174 mg) of cholesterol, and keep in mind that .003 oz (100 mg) daily mean 5 more points added to the cholesterol level in the blood. According to this example, the fillet would mean almost 9 points more added. And this number can go much higher if we add sausages, fast food, hot dogs, and many products containing animal fat. These "saturated" fats are completely different to those that come from vegetable oils, or "unsaturated" fats, which do not contain cholesterol. However, keep in mind that palm or coconut oil or hydrogenated oils (like margarine) are high in saturated fats.

On the other hand, vegetable products such as grains, legumes, fruits, vegetables, seeds, sprouts, plant-based proteins, algae, and others are completely devoid of cholesterol and their fat content is very low or null in some cases.

Hydrogenated oils are often used in industrial pastries, cakes, and cookies. Read product labels before buying, especially if you are overweight.

Atherosclerosis is a disorder that can begin at an early age, although it takes time to develop.

The shift toward this type of diet helps arterial blockages to clear out naturally. If this cleansing process is not done, the next step is to face one of the most common heart diseases, atherosclerosis.

ATHEROSCLEROSIS

This disease occurs when there is an accumulation of fat and cholesterol formations that enter the artery walls reducing its elasticity. So this disease is also known as "hardening of the arteries." Cholesterol in our food doubles our risk for atherosclerosis, according to research on this matter.

HDL AND LDL

Most health articles often refer to this acronym. One of them represents good cholesterol (HDL), and the other represents bad cholesterol (LDL). Here we need to clarify one point: this is not about foods having good cholesterol; HDL is considered good because the body can eliminate it. HDL, *high density lipoprotein*, consists of large molecules that our body uses for its elimination.

When HDL level is low, it means that we need to elevate it. What can we do? Eating foods that contain antioxidants and physical exercise helps to increase HDL levels. By contrast, excess weight and smoking bring it down.

LDL, *low density lipoprotein,* is the "bad cholesterol," a small molecule that can penetrate arterial walls and form so-called "fat lines."

Another word much used in reference to heart problems is "triglycerides." Which are fat molecules that form in the liver and travel through the blood. A high level of triglycerides puts us at risk for heart disease. To keep it at bay, exercise and follow a diet that is low in fat and sugar, since those foods can also raise it. Today it is very easy to get tested to know your triglyceride and cholesterol levels in the blood. There are many pharmacies that offer this service.

"BAD" FATS

Some time ago, when the effects of saturated fats on health came to be known, many people switched from butter to margarine because, they said, margarine is a plant product and it does not increase cholesterol. Recently, margarine was found to also be a saturated fat. But how is that possible, if it comes from a vegetable source? Vegetable oil that margarine is made from is manipulated so that it stays solid at room temperature. This process requires that hydrogen be injected at high pressure and temperature, and in so doing approximately 25% of nonsatured fats become semisaturated hydrogenated fats.

Pastries with less fat

If you have to bake cakes, cookies, or pastries, replace butter or margarine in recipes with mashed prunes. To make it, shred 5 oz (140 g) pitted prunes with six tablespoons of water.

Spectacular Superfoods

In addition, hydrogenation converts another 25% more fat into "trans fats," the famous "trans acids." Recent studies have found that these fats are as harmful, if not more, than saturated fats. About seven years ago, a group of researchers from Denmark found that high doses of trans fats further reduced HDL and increased LDL in the blood. But it is not all bad news: there are margarines made with non-hydrogenated oil, such as organic ones.

SUPERFOODS FOR THE HEART

These foods help lower cholesterol or protect the heart from disorders that may occur over time. Hawthorn (*Crataegus oxicanta*) and cayenne pepper also help keep you in peak condition.

•**Avocado**. It is very rich in monounsaturated fat, and can increase HDL cholesterol and lower LDL. It's always better not eat too much of it because it has a lot of calories.

•**Garlic**. Thousands of years ago Dioscorides said that garlic cured arteries. Medical journals continuously publish scientific evidence that verifies it. In the 1970s R. C. Jain, University of Benghazi, Libya, showed that garlic prevents the formation of plaque in the arteries and helps prevent atherosclerosis and heart disease. Other studies certify that it acts against hypertension, helps reduce LDL cholesterol, and increases HDL. All it takes is one raw garlic clove a day.

• **Beans**. Eating a cup of cooked beans every day can reduce the rate of cholesterol by ten percent. Beans are also rich in folic acid, which regulates the concentration of the amino acid homocysteine in the body. High levels of this substance in the blood can be as bad for the heart as smoking.

• **Foods with antioxidants**. Foods rich in beta carotene and vitamins C and E play a special role: protect cholesterol particles from damage as they travel through the blood. And why do they do that? Because damaged cholesterol particles (by free radicals) end up being absorbed by the artery wall and start to form plaques that impede blood flow.

•**Celery.** In celery stalk there is a compound (3-n-butyl phthalide) that gives it its characteristic aroma and can help control blood pressure. Eating four celery stalks daily can reduce cholesterol by fourteen percent.

• **Olive oil.** It is an important part of the Mediterranean diet and luckily for us, it is not only delicious but it is also a monounsaturated fat. Virgin olive oil is the best source of essential fatty acids that lower LDL and increase HDL. To make sure you have a high quality product, make sure it is extra virgin, cold pressed, and organic.

Pectin found in apples forms a gel that absorbs LDL cholesterol and helps eliminate toxins.

• **Fiber.** Soluble fiber found in many foods lowers cholesterol levels. Among foods most recommended for their fiber to prevent atherosclerosis are legumes, oats, barley, vegetables, and fruit.

• **Pu-erh tea.** This tea originates from China and rose to fame when a group of doctors from Kunming Institute of Medicine gave evidence that it reduced cholesterol levels in the blood. It also reduces triglycerides and elevated fat levels in the blood. Three cups a day will give excellent results as long as bad habits causing the problem are monitored.

• **Green Tea.** Harvard University endorses it. According to their research, a couple of cups a day may reduce the risk of stroke by 45%. Its strength lies in bioflavonoids, the substance that gives antioxidant power.

• **Lemon.** In addition to improving arterial elasticity, drinking lemon juice, with its rind, is a good treatment for hypercholesterolemia since it has citroflavonoids in its bark and contains pectin in the flavedo (the white part beneath the skin). Research shows that it lowers LDL cholesterol by forty percent.

• **Nuts.** According to data published by the British Medical Journal, eating nuts is associated to a significant reduction in cardiovascular disease. They are also effective at reducing high cholesterol levels when eaten in place of animal fats. They are antioxidant (vitamin E and carotenoids). A daily serving of five nuts is enough.

• **Grapes.** Its flavonoids and antioxidants keep blood clots from forming and prevent atherosclerosis.

• **Soy.** Soy is one of the best replacements of animal protein and it has the added advantage that it contains no fat or cholesterol. Its derivative, lecithin, is recommended for regulating cholesterol. It also helps digestion and absorption of fats and fat-soluble vitamins.

HELPFUL DIETARY SUPPLEMENTS

• **Garlic capsules.** If you cannot stand raw garlic, you can opt for garlic oil extract in gel capsules. Besides regulating cholesterol levels, it has vasodilatory properties that promote good cardiovascular function.

• **B Vitamins.** This group of vitamins (B6, B9 or folic acid, and B12) helps reduce the risk of heart attacks by controlling homocysteine level in the blood, which is an amino acid that accelerates hardening of the arteries (atherosclerosis).

• **Coenzyme Q$_{10}$.** Also called "Vitamin Q," it is a substance that our body makes and is present in many foods such as broccoli, nuts, and spinach. It is also possible to find it as a supplement for heart conditions. It has been

Antioxidants foods strengthen the heart

• **Beta-carotene.** Yellow and orange fruits and vegetables (carrot, apricot, peach, melon) and spinach and parsley.

• **Vitamin C.** Citrus, red pepper, kiwi, strawberries, berries, and broccoli.

• **Vitamin E.** Wheat germ, sunflower seeds and whole grains.

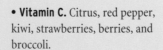
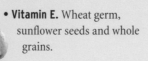

used successfully to treat cardiomyopathy, heart failure, congestive heart disease, and atherosclerosis. In Denmark, patients on a wait list for heart transplant showed such significant improvement of myocardial contractility after taking this supplement that they no longer needed the transplant. It also tends to be very effective while taking medication to lower LDL cholesterol, since these drugs inhibit the production of Q_{10} that the body produces.

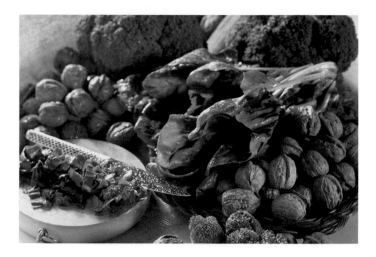

- **Green tea capsules.** If you do not have time to enjoy a cup of this tea (which you should try to do), there are capsules containing its active ingredients.

- **Soy lecithin.** It is highly recommended for its hypocholesterolemic action (lowers LDL and increases HDL). It is available as granules and capsules.

- **L-carnitine.** This is an amino acid that stimulates metabolism of fats. It helps reduce triglycerides and LDL cholesterol, and increases energy. In general, it improves cardiac function.

- **Evening primrose oil and borage oil.** Both are sources of GLA (gamma-linoleic acid), which is an "essential" fatty acid because the body does not produce it and must

get it from food. They help the heart by reducing LDL cholesterol and preventing blood platelets from sticking together to form clots. It is believed that maximum effects are achieved after three months of regularly taking evening primrose oil or borage oil in terms of lowering cholesterol. The percentages vary depending on individual eating habits.

Pay attention to excess iron!

Eating too much red meat increases iron and cholesterol levels. Excess iron can increase the risk of heart disease, because it acts as a catalyst for the production of free radicals that can damage cholesterol, facilitating the formation of plaques.

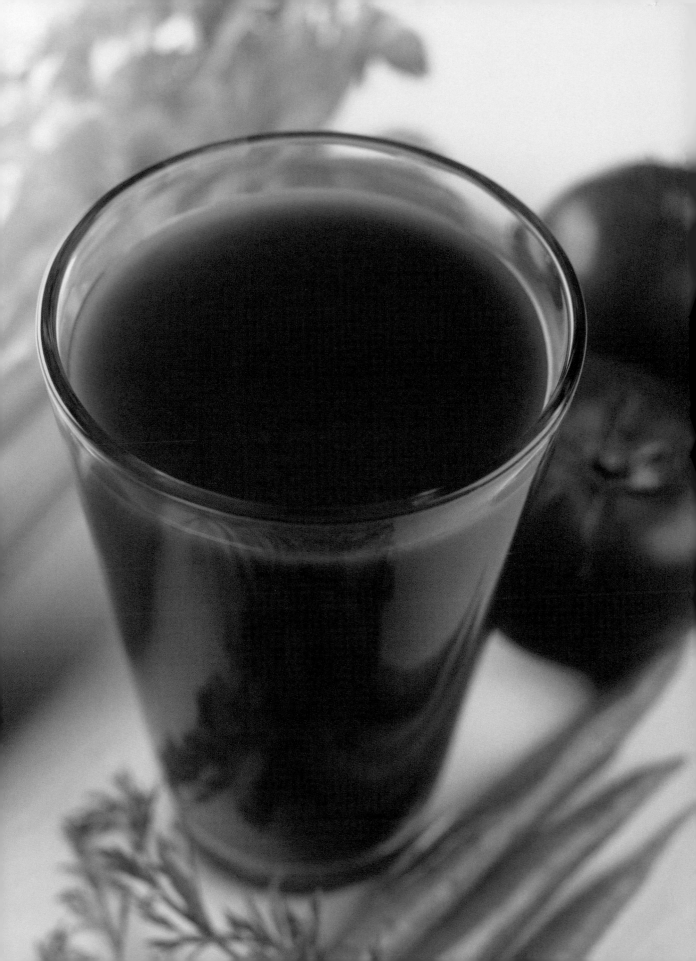

Food combinations

4

How to combine food

Food compatibility charts

Eat everything . . . but not all at once (food and weight control)

Living without heartburn: The delicate balance between enzymes

How to combine food

Would you drink a glass of milk with vinegar? Of course not, they obviously do not mix well; that is, they are not compatible. As we will see in this chapter, there are a number of foods that do not go well with each other.

The quality of a diet depends not only on choosing fresh and healthy food, but also how they mix. Randomly mixing foods may complicate digestion and health, and will sometimes cancel out their benefits.

When we overload the digestive system, we are taking energy away from the body that could be used for more beneficial purposes. In that sense, we must pay special attention to the compatibility of food to avoid energy deficiency, and know which **nutritional associations** are especially significant. Let us first see how what we eat is combined in the digestive tract. We will first take a look at wonderful natural fermenting agents: enzymes.

• **Ptyalin.** It is secreted in the mouth and converts starches into disaccharides such as maltose and sucrose. It acts only in a moderately alkaline reaction, since a too alkaline reaction or an acidic reaction destroys this enzyme.

• **Pepsin.** It is secreted in the stomach and pancreas, where it transforms fat into fatty acids. It requires an acidic environment to act, whereas an alkaline environment immediately destroys it. It is also suppressed by very cold foods such as ice cream and drinks.

• **Amylase.** It is found in the stomach and liver. It transforms the fats in food into fatty acids that can be absorbed by the bloodstream.

• **Lipase.** It is found in the stomach and liver. It transforms the fats in food into fatty acids that can be absorbed by the bloodstream.

• **Renin.** Children secrete it in the stomach until about age seven. It acts on casein, which is responsible for coagulating milk.

INCOMPATIBLE COMBINATIONS

Acidic foods and starches should not be included in the same meal because acidic foods destroy ptyalin, an enzyme needed to digest starches. Starches also take longer to digest than fruit, hindering the entire digestive process. In short, eat acidic foods by themselves and separate from other types of food.

Likewise, do not combine proteins (especially defatted protein, such as yogurt or kefir) with concentrated starches (bread, rice, starches), as they each have different digestive processes.

Combinations in the digestive tract

• Enzymes (or natural fermenting agents) participate in food digestion. They break down food into simple nutrients: lipids into fatty acids, proteins into amino acids, starches into glucose . . . Afterward, the nutrients enter into the bloodstream to feed the cells.

• Different types of enzymes have different functions. Each enzyme acts on food substances in a particular way.

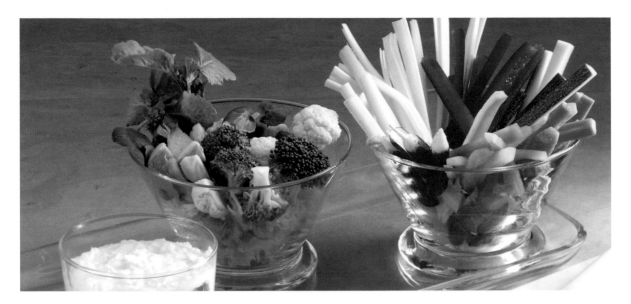

This means avoiding some classic sandwiches, unless they are made with whole wheat bread mixed with proteins like cheese, mayonnaise, or egg.

Sugars (added or naturally present in fruit) ferment in the stomach when there is starch. This happens because each of these foods is digested differently. So, fruit cupcakes (especially if they contain highly acidic fruit) and toast with jam are particularly incompatible (indigestible). If you cannot resist eating cupcakes, do not eat them with a main meal to avoid such fermentation. Another option is to eat them before a meal, since they are quickly digested.

Milk combines poorly with other food categories, except as cottage cheese, yogurt, or kefir with acidic fruit. Finally, it should be noted that nature intended milk for infants and children, because after age seven we no longer have renin, the enzyme that allows us to absorb all of milk's nutrients.

MODERATELY COMPATIBLE COMBINATIONS

Fats combine fairly well with starches, as the first slow decomposition of the latter.

A lengthier digestive process allows gastric juices to better absorb different foods. These combinations are generally good unless the person suffers from energy deficiency.

Moderately compatible

• Grains + legumes: beans and rice, veggie crepes, etc.
• Grains + egg or cheese: bread and cheese, bread and boiled egg with mayonnaise, etc.
• Starches + egg or cheese or legumes: beans and potatoes, squash and carrot with grated cheese, potatoes with aioli, etc.
• Legumes + seeds: humus (chickpeas with sesame), vegetable soup with sunflower seeds, etc.

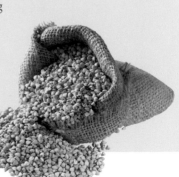

As for proteins, avoid combining two different types because they each will likely have a different digestive process. Also avoid combining protein with fat, unless the latter makes up a small proportion of the plate. Fat reduces gastric secretion and inhibits pepsin, the enzyme responsible for transforming proteins into amino acids.

Sugars and proteins should be eaten separately, since sugars are only digested in the intestine. However, in some cases they mix fairly well.

Finally, combining two different starches (for example, rice and potatoes) is not optimal, so it is best for the body to digest them separately. The most compatible are logically those that are closest. In that sense, good combinations include grains or purees made with potatoes, squash, and carrot.

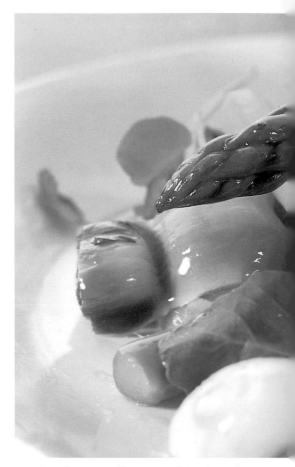

Fairly good combinations

Monosaccharide + fat protein: tahini with apple, apple with Burgos cheese, etc.
• Monosaccharide + lean protein: dairy + fruit, dried fruit + dairy, etc.

• Disaccharide + protein: nuts (previously soaked) with yogurt, kefir, cottage cheese, etc.

COMPATIBLE COMBINATIONS

Fruits combine well with each other as long as we do not mix very sweet varieties with others that are highly acidic (banana + lemon, fig + orange).

Meanwhile, proteins and vegetables combine perfectly, since they require similar digestion processes. Vegetables also provide water and minerals that facilitate protein absorption.

Another excellent combination is starch and vegetables, as the latter facilitate digestion of the former. This happy union includes dishes like vegetable and rice paella with a green salad.

Starches also mix remarkably well with fats, resulting in interesting dishes like potatoes with olive oil, avocado and potato salad, and so on. Fats also mix well with vegetables, since fats moderately slow the digestion of vegetables.

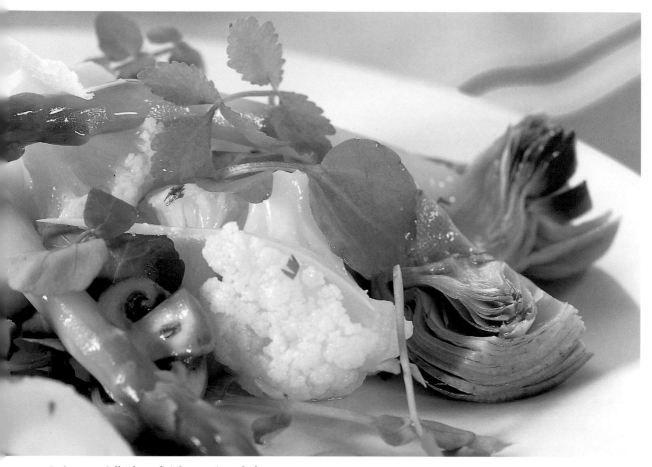

It is especially beneficial to mix salads or steamed vegetables with cold-pressed extra virgin olive oil and then add pine nuts or walnuts.

HOW MUCH SHOULD WE EAT?

Although amounts may vary slightly, inactive adults are recommended to eat 53 oz (1500 g) of food per day, of which 17 oz (500 g) should be dry; active adults are recommended to eat up to 84 oz (2400 g) of food per day, of which 28 oz (800 g) should be dry.

With a whole grain diet, it is best to spread out food into small meals throughout the day instead of "feasting." For children

The Best Combinations

- Sweet fruits + sweet fruits (e.g. banana and apple)
- Sweet fruits + semi-acid fruits (e.g. cherry and apple)
- Semi-acid fruits + semi-acid fruits (e.g. peach and cherry)

and adolescents, the ideal diet consists of around 4 or 6 daily meals, 3 or 4 meals for healthy adults, and 2 or 3 meals for the elderly.

FOOD COMPATIBILITY CHART

Carbohydrates

Legend

Positive — Applies to all energy situations

■ **Neutral** — Use cautiously in case of energy deficiency

▲ **Incompatible** — Avoid at all times

Simple sugars / Double sugars — food lists

Acidic	Semi-acidic	Sweet	Dried	Neutral	Honey	Double sugars
Kiwi, Orange, Lemon, Mandarin, Tangerine, Grapefruit, Tomato, Pomegranate, Pineapple, Grapefruit, Currant, Mango, Blueberry	Cherry, Apricots, Plum, Papaya, Strawberry, Sour pear, Sour peach, Sour apple, Nectarine	Fresh date, Fresh figs, Sweet grape, Golden or Russet apple, Plantain, Banana, Banana, Quince, Cherry, Rhubarb	Raisin, Currant, Prune, Date, Dried figs, Dried apricots	Cantaloupe, Watermelon	Honey of all kinds	Brown sugar, Powder sugar, Beet sugar, Apple syrup, Marmalade, Jam, Royal jelly, Honeyed fruit, Candied fruit

Compatibility matrix

Category		Acidic	Semi-acidic	Sweet	Dried	Neutral	Honey	Double sugars
Carbohydrates — Simple sugars	Acidic			■	■	■	■	■
	Semi-acidic					■		■
	Sweet	■				■		
	Dried	■				■	■	■
	Neutral	■	■	■	■		■	■
	Honey	■			■	■	■	
Carbohydrates	Double sugars	■	■	■	■	■	■	
	Starches	▲	▲	▲	■	▲	■	▲
Proteins	Legumes	▲	▲	▲	▲	▲	▲	▲
	Lean protein	■				■	■	■
	Fat protein	■	■	▲	■	■	■	▲
Milk		▲	▲	▲	▲	▲	▲	▲
Lipids		▲	▲	■	▲	▲	■	■
Vegetables	Weak starch	■	▲	■	■	▲	■	▲
	Mild starch	▲	▲	▲	▲	▲	▲	▲
Water		■	■	■	▲	■	■	
Salt		▲	▲	▲	▲	▲	▲	

Starches	Protein			Milk	Lipids	Vegetables		Water	Salt
	Legumes	Lean protein	Protein			Weak starch	Mild starch		

Starches	Legumes	Lean protein	Protein	Lipids	Weak starch	Mild starch
Grains	Green soybeans	Yoghurt	Fatty cheese	Oils	Asparagus	Pepper
Oats	Red soy or adzuki beans	Sour milk	Emmental cheese	Olive	Cooked broccoli	Beet
Wheat	Yellow soybeans	Fresh cheese	Gruyere	Sunflower	Cooked eggplant	Carrot
Corn	Lentils	Cottage cheese	Comté cheese	Soy	Cucumber	Cabbage
Rye	Fava beans	Kefir	Manchego with low-salt	Defatted corn	Zucchini	Brussels sprouts
Barley	String beans	Nonó	Meat	Grapeseed	Watercress	Parsley
Millet	Kidney beans	Dry brewer's yeast	Oils	Peanut	Endive	Garlic
Buckwheat	Peas	Torula yeast	Almond	Safflower	Raw spinach	Squash
Brown rice	Grass peas	Goat cheese	Hazelnut	Cream	Lettuce	Kohlrabi
Starches	Vetch	Acidic cheese	Walnut	Butter	Escarole	Parsnip
Potato	Chickpeas	Sprouts	Pine nut	Avocado	Sorrel	Thistle
Sweet potato	Alfalfa	Fish	Pistachio	Margarine	Red cabbage	Onion
Tapioca			Olive	Mayonnaise	Mushroom	Garlic
Flour, pasta and semolina			Peanut	Aioli	Chard	Leek
			Egg	Coconut	Celery	Turnip
						Raw cabbage
						Dandelion

Food combinations

In any case, more or less intuitively, we all know that some foods, combined with others, are more tasty, healthy, or nutritious. A plate of salad is a good example of this: when vegetables are eaten separately, they may taste quite bland, but when you mix them and add good olive oil, salt or gomasio (ground sesame seeds with sea salt) and some tamari (soy sauce) or vinegar, they become a delicious dish. By contrast, other foods that are very healthy and nutritious when eaten by themselves may be indigestible when combined.

Since the nineteenth century, doctors and dietitians have aimed to study what makes foods compatible or incompatible. This type of research is complex, because we are not likely to agree on one single universal criterion.

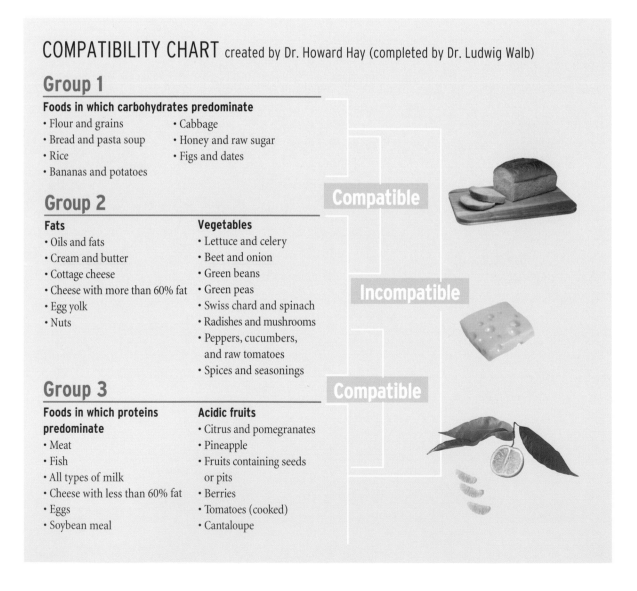

COMPATIBILITY CHART created by Dr. Howard Hay (completed by Dr. Ludwig Walb)

Group 1
Foods in which carbohydrates predominate
- Flour and grains
- Bread and pasta soup
- Rice
- Bananas and potatoes
- Cabbage
- Honey and raw sugar
- Figs and dates

Group 2
Fats
- Oils and fats
- Cream and butter
- Cottage cheese
- Cheese with more than 60% fat
- Egg yolk
- Nuts

Vegetables
- Lettuce and celery
- Beet and onion
- Green beans
- Green peas
- Swiss chard and spinach
- Radishes and mushrooms
- Peppers, cucumbers, and raw tomatoes
- Spices and seasonings

Group 3
Foods in which proteins predominate
- Meat
- Fish
- All types of milk
- Cheese with less than 60% fat
- Eggs
- Soybean meal

Acidic fruits
- Citrus and pomegranates
- Pineapple
- Fruits containing seeds or pits
- Berries
- Tomatoes (cooked)
- Cantaloupe

Compatible

Incompatible

Compatible

Our nutrition is affected by which foods we eat, the **condition** foods are in when we eat them, and our health. No matter how healthy a dish is, if you eat in a hurry, with **nervousness** or anxiety, it may end up making you feel bad.

Moreover, compatibility depends largely on the **amount** that we put on our plate (almost as much as the substances it contains). "With small portions, there are no incompatibilities," as the famous naturopath Dr. Eduardo Alfonso would say.

As shown in the previous tables, eggs and potatoes are incompatible, and yet they are part of many dishes. Are we to give up eating, for example, fried eggs with potatoes? Not at all. We just need to reduce the amount of one of these two ingredients and refrain from eating them often, since they are not very recommended, especially if you want to lose some pounds.

Another key element to avoid food incompatibilities—and to better digest and absorb food—is drinking at mealtimes. They say that most people who start their meal by eating salads or raw foods enjoy better digestion and do not feel as thirsty during their meal. To help digestion, **avoid drinking liquids** while eating.

So, a good diet is based on selecting compatible food groups. Avoid mixing too many ingredients, if at all possible.

Do you want proof? This is an easy way to check: you will for sure have eaten churros ("fritters") with chocolate for breakfast or as a snack. And surely, after a few bites you start to feel stuffed. The explanation is simple: besides having refried oil, churros have a lot of incompatibilities: sugar, oil, potatoes, flour, etc.

Is "compatibility" the same as "combination"?

No, although both are closely related concepts from a dietary point of view. Food compatibility depends on the nature of their nutrients and their relationship with our body during digestion.

Combination refers to the possibilities certain foods offer for a specific purpose, such as weight loss or nutrient supplementation during an illness.

Remember that vague feeling of lethargy that keeps you from being able to focus and makes you want to take a short nap is not a sign of good digestion, it indicates precisely the opposite: an extra effort in the stomach and liver. This type of indigestion is more or less bearable, but it can cause problems over time. It is not good to mix foods randomly no matter how much we like certain ingredients.

Doctors Howard Hay and Ludwig Walb have carefully studied food digestibility and compatibility. So far, their conclusions (shown in the table on the previous page) have become the most reliable and widespread when planning a diet.

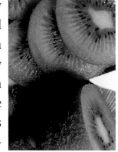

Acidic fruits like kiwi, are often very nutritious but less compatible than others.

Eat everything . . . but not all at once (food and weight control)

More recently, the "dissociated diet" has garnered, with some variations, a major success. The reason is simple: it helps us to **naturally control our weight** and obesity.

Such diets are based on cleverly combining food, which we summarize in the table on the next page. We all know the importance of preventing disorders caused by food, such as anorexia or bulimia, and in general, all health problems stemming from excess weight because in developed societies we have a tendency to eat inorganic, refined, processed foods with little nutritional value, in large amounts and at odd times of the day. One of the first to realize all this was Michel Montignac, who due to his profession, had to attend many business lunches that were overloaded with fat and salt, processed, or cooked again and again in microwave ovens . . . He was one of the first to realize that the best thing to do is:

• Drink water upon waking.
• Eat a good breakfast.
• Have mid-morning snack.
• Drink a glass of water before eating.
• Start lunch with a salad. Leave fruit (one piece) for a snack.
• Drink another glass of water before dinner.
• Start dinner with a plate of raw foods.
• Drink a relaxing tea two hours after dinner.

Living without heartburn: The delicate balance between enzymes

Enzymes act on a different type of food and to be able to act, they need a certain environment, which are important good food combinations.

• **Ptyalin.** It is segregated in the salivary glands and acts on the starches (predigestion). However, it is an enzyme that is easily destroyed when there is heartburn (acid or very alkaline pH). Therefore, do not eat grains or starches in general, with meat or acidic fruit.

• **Amylase.** It is segregated in the salivary glands and pancreas, and acts on starches and carbohydrates in general.

• **Pepsin.** It is secreted in the stomach and acts on starches and carbohydrates. It is active in acidity (it is immediately destroyed in an alkaline). It is interrupted by sudden temperature change (for example, a cold drink).

• **Lipase.** It is secreted by the pancreas and metabolizes fats, turning them into fatty acids.

THREE FOOD GROUPS

Protein group	Neutral group	Starch group
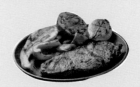	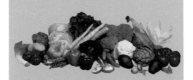	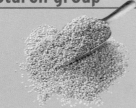

Protein group

- Any type of meat
- Sausages
- Beef broth

- Any type of fish
- Crustaceans
- Mollusks

- Eggs

- Milk, cheese and yogurt

- Legumes
- Green peas
- Fava beans
- Kidney beans
- Lentils
- Soya and derivatives

Neutral group

All vegetables except legumes
- Seeds
- Nuts
- Almonds
- Hazelnuts
- Sesame seeds

- Olive oil
- Seed oil
- Salt
- Herbs and spices

Starch group

All grains and derivatives
- Oats
- Spelt
- Wheat
- Corn
- Millet
- Rye
- Rice
- Barley
- Flour
- Bread
- Pasta
- Corn cakes

- Potatoes

Foods in this group:

- Can be combined with neutral foods (green group).

- Cannot be combined with starches (blue group).

- Cannot be combined with each other.

Foods in this group:

- Can be combined with protein foods (orange group).

- Can be combined with starches (blue group).

- Can be combined with each other.

Foods in this group:

- Can be combined with neutral foods (green group).

- Can be combined with each other.

- Can be combined with proteins (orange group)

Food combinations

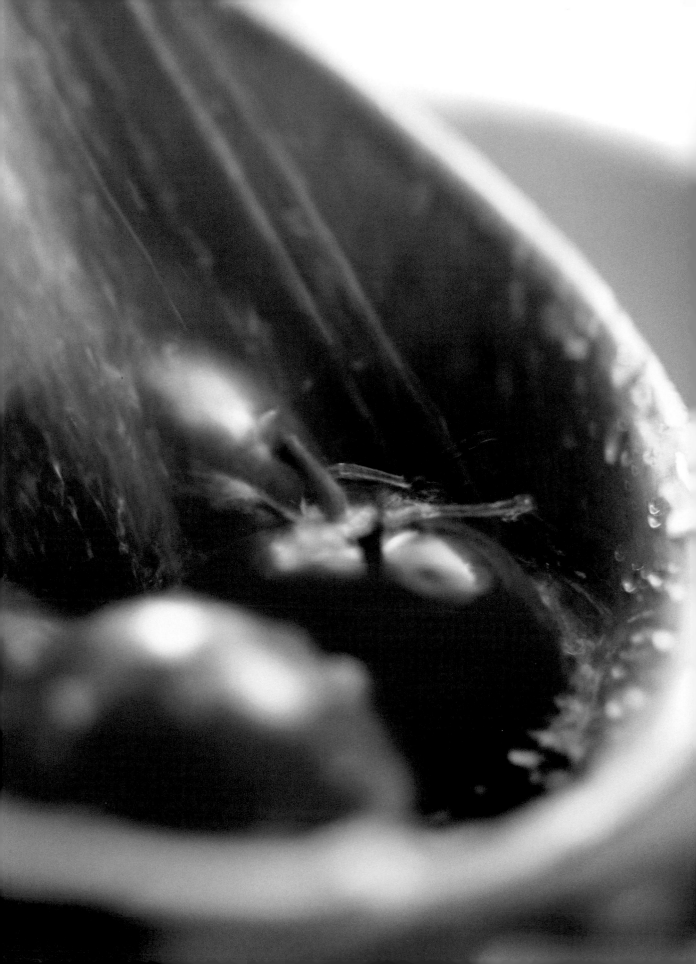

Utensils and cooking techniques

5 Food preservation
Preparing food
Cooking utensils

You can retrain your palate with delicious, healthy flavors, both new and forgotten.

Fine cuisine with abundant flavors, does not have to be at odds with good health, as we are learning. We will prepare tasty and nutritious menus, using classic and new cuisines.

Once we understand the necessary nutrients, and which foods and superfoods are preferable, it's time to plan meals and start working in the kitchen. In this chapter we review a few essential tips, to preserve and prepare food without spoiling it. As we know, any product, from harvest to the table, goes through a process of collection, distribution, marketing, and preparation with hygiene and conservation; but unfortunately, due to changes in the market and society, fruits, vegetables, and legumes which are harvested unripe, lose a substantial part of their flavor and nutritional content. However, it is worth remembering the ten rules of the World Health Organization (WHO) on food handling that concern us all:

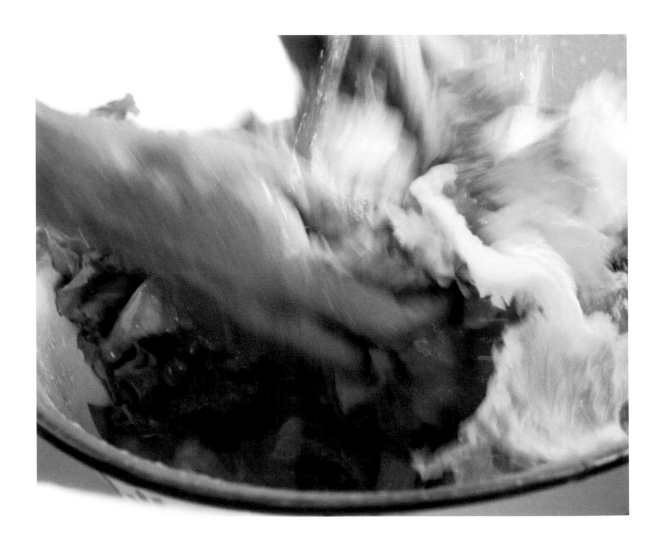

1. Always choose foods treated in the least aggressive way possible. Fruits, vegetables, and legumes do not require special treatment at home before eating. But, for example, oranges are washed with chemicals and waxed to appear shinier; legumes are treated to prevent molding . . . and this list is endless for "natural" foods, which cease to be wholesome and become potentially dangerous. Hence the importance of buying organic food (without pesticides or synthetic chemical additives) which go directly from the orchard to the store. Sometimes they are more expensive and less attractive, but they are definitely healthier. It has been said that fertilizers and genetic engineering make plastic wonders.

As for milk, although it is more nutritious raw, it is safest to get pasteurized milk to avoid germs that can cause disorders and diseases.

2. Cook food thoroughly as needed. All fruits and many vegetables can be eaten raw, but there are a few foods that require heat. Safe temperature is 158° F (70° C) and all parts of the food must reach this temperature.

3. Eat freshly cooked food as soon as possible. Although cooking kills most microorganisms—and, unfortunately, many nutrients—microbes can still proliferate in food, so eat right away.

Pasteurization and homogenization

Milk cartons often read "pasteurized and homogenized," which are two treatments that raw milk undergoes to preserve it in a safe manner. Pasteurization involves heating milk to 149° F (65° C) and cooled sharply to 39.2° F (4° C) several times to remove all bacteria.

Homogenization involves the injection of steam at 266 or 284° F (130 or 140° C) for two to three seconds and reducing the temperature to 158° F (70° C). Thus, the fat globules are broken down, preventing the milk from coagulating.

4. Store raw or cooked food appropriately. Foods that are exposed to temperatures between 41° F (5° C) and 158° F (70° C) begin to degrade, so you have to store them in the refrigerator immediately.

5. Reheat cooked foods at about 158° F (70° C). It is always preferable to avoid reheating food more than once.

6. Avoid contact between raw food and cooked food. All these guidelines would be useless if cooked food and raw food are stored together (particularly if it is not properly cleaned).

7. Keep your hands clean at all times.

8. Keep the kitchen clean. Before and after cooking, thoroughly wash all work surfaces and utensils that are to be used. You can also add a few drops of bleach to the water and then rinse thoroughly.

The WHO's 10 rules in summary:
- Cleaning
- Monitoring cooking time and temperatures
- Proper conservation

Utensils and cooking techniques

9. Protect food from animals. This refers to pets (keep dog or cat food from coming into contact with other foods) as well as rodents and insects.

10. Always use clean water. Cooking with unclean water, even when it is boiled, can cause food poisoning. Moreover, more and more consumers avoid tap water and cook using bottled or filtered water.

Food preservation

Over time, no food remains intact due to enzymatic reactions or the growth of microorganisms.

To prevent degradation there are several types of conservation that yield good results. Still, we insist on the importance of choosing the most nutritional food possible, avoiding canned (smoked, cured, and salted).

• **Using a double boiler.** Fruits, vegetables, and legumes can be kept in sealed containers and heated to a certain temperature to eliminate degrading enzymes, germs, and toxins. They can be prepared at home following traditional rules.

• **Dehydration.** It consists of air drying foods to rid them of their water content. In doing so, microorganisms will not have the means to develop. It is one of the oldest methods for preserving foods. It is done using vacuum seals.

• **Refrigeration and freezing.** Germs develop at a certain temperature. To avoid it, keep food cold. For their immediate use, temperature should be between 35.6° F (2° C) and 41° F (5° C). For freezing, food must reach -11.2° F (-24° C). Frozen foods keep better but they tend to produce thirst as they are digested.

Beware of irradiated food!

Developed in the early 1950s, it eliminates insects and microorganisms from fruits, vegetables, and grains and delaying it from ripening, which in principle could be considered an advantage, as it allows more time for transport and storage. However, the presence of radioactive isotopes in food (even when below 1 mrad, the maximum accepted) cannot have good consequences on our health.

Preparing food

The secret in good natural cooking and almost every cuisine lies on three principles: a good selection of food, good preparation, and good presentation. In this book we discuss food, the best portion sizes for our daily diet, and nutritional value. It is time to turn to some cooking techniques that we should know well.

Anyone who wants to become a good cook must learn to peel, cut, grind. . . . These are basic culinary techniques but there are other, more complex involving more tools (straining, filtering, boiling, frying . . .). If you are interested in learning more ways of preparing and cooking styles, you will find such information in the final pages of this book.

on the direction in which cuts are made, as well as the thickness and texture of the pieces. It is essential to have a good set of sharp knives. To cut vegetables, you need to have a knife with a sharp tip, which comes in handy when cutting thick skin of certain vegetables such as squash, watermelon, and cantaloupe.

Chinese knives that are blunt and rectangular can cut vegetables faster and though they are increasingly easier to find, they can be replaced with pastry or cheese knives. Special knives are for cutting certain foods and make decorative cuts.

PEEL

Generally, we use a small knife that can be handled well, with a tip and a cutting edge that is sharp enough to separate the outermost layer of fruits or vegetables. If you do not have a lot of time or too much skill, use a peeler, an instrument quite similar to a knife with a curved blade and a sharp cleft in its center.

New manual large potato peelers are very useful also for peeling carrots with great comfort, especially if they are not organically grown.

CUT

Cutting food is one of the most important steps in cooking, since flavor and consistency of the dish can vary significantly depending

You need to master culinary techniques to get the most out of your food.

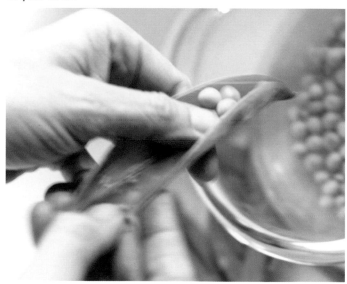

Is it better to cook with wood and clay tools?

Sometimes we hear high praise for "artisanal" bread cooked with firewood or maybe we get excited when we get to use aluminum pots. But we do not know if there are real benefits to applying these traditional methods. So to find out whether it is better to cook with firewood and use glazed clay or materials, we will review some research that tries to scientifically explain these preferences. Above all, there is no doubt that the quality of water when cooking also depends on the source of heat as well as the container used.

Source of heat affects water quality

The experiment was done as follows: distilled water was boiled in a reflux condenser using different fuels: gas, electricity, coal, wood, and straw.

For 20 minutes water remained boiling and then it was cooled to 62.6° F (17° C). The water was then used for germinating wheat: grains were left to germinate in porcelain containers with water. After 10 days the length of the leaves was measured and the measurements of the roots were used to produce graphs on fuel quality.

The result was very significant: for leaf length, electricity is a less favorable heat source, followed by gas, coal, firewood, and straw. Electricity and gas have a very marked inhibitory effect compared to the control (distilled water), while wood and straw instead have a stimulating effect.

In this regard, it is interesting to note that modern heating appliances are worse than straw (mixed with dirt or cow dung), which is used commonly in poor countries.

Physicists claim that a calorie is always a calorie, regardless of their origin, but this experiment clearly demonstrates that there are different qualities of heat and more traditional methods offer greater reliability in terms of said quality. Not to mention today's microwave ovens that warm up food at the molecular level using electromagnetic waves that are capable of penetrating containers.

Containers affect water quality

A similar test was done to test whether the material that container was made of affected the water that was boiled in it. The procedure was the same: water was boiled for 20 minutes in aluminum, iron, tin, copper, glass, enamel, porcelain, earthenware, and gold containers.

The water was cooled to 62.6° F (17° C) and used to make wheat germinate. The lengths of the leaves and roots after 10 days also yielded some clear results since considerable differences in growth were observed depending on the container used. Again the most modern materials are the worst (aluminum is the most harmful).

Gold is at the top, which may seem surprising, given that other metals are at the other end of the spectrum. We must take into account the value attributed to gold by all civilizations that have known this metal's sacred value. Unlike today, for ancient civilizations, gold was not only a precious metal because of its rarity; no doubt, its attributed value was much due to the fact that they recognized its outstanding properties, as this experiment confirms. Immediately after gold comes earthenware, which is made

with one of the simplest and oldest materials known.

A practical conclusion would be that it is better to use earthenware (1) or enameled (2) containers *as much as possible*. As for cooking with wood, it is certainly not very comfortable, but it is better than gas, coal, or electric appliances.

It is true that "human beings are not wheat grains" but the fact remains that there are universal biological laws.

* According to research done by R. Hauschka.

Aluminum tools are not recommended because minimal (although harmful) amounts of aluminum dissolve in foods, which can cause metabolic imbalances. Acidic foods can dissolve aluminum when it is heated. Vinegar with salt can be dangerous with aluminum, as well as hot fruit juices and, ultimately, any food that contains a combination of salt and acid. So, if you are using aluminum cookware avoid cookings our fruits, tomatoes, milk, and never add salt or baking to foods that are being cooked.

(1) We do not know any manufacturer of gold pots, but the difference in quality between gold and clay does not justify the price difference.
(2) Some materials used in ceramic glazes are poisonous, particularly the compounds with lead. To avoid this, ceramic industries (under current standards throughout Europe) perform different processes. For example, vitrified ceramic ("Bisbal" pottery) has a lead sulfide coating, which once mixed with quartz becomes insoluble silicate lead. In almost every country there are safety standards for ceramic glazes.

The best known are perhaps those that pierce cylindrical forms; that can be used to hollow apples, potatoes, etc. or to fill them. Although they are very useful, they can always be replaced with a sharp knife and a spoon.

To cut comfortably you need a good unvarnished wooden board measuring about 12 inches (30 cm) long and 8 inches (20 cm) high and about 1 or 1.5 inches (3 or 4 cm) thick. It must be of good quality, because it will be used and washed daily. Beech and pine woods, with few veins, are best.

GRATE

Graters allow us to crumble foods such as carrots, bread, eggs, or cheese, for example.

The best are rectangular single use graters (those with grooves on one side going in one direction). Those made from stainless steel can be kept for long. The ideal would be to have two: one with medium grooves for vegetables, fruits, eggs, etc., and one with small grooves for nutmeg, cheese, bread, almonds, and other foods of similar hardness and texture.

There are other more complex interchangeable graters that are electric, have interchangeable disks, or operate with a hand crank. They can be handled much more easily than others, but some cannot withstand too much pressure and tend to break. They also tend not to grate very finely.

A cutting board made out of beech or pine will be very useful in the kitchen.

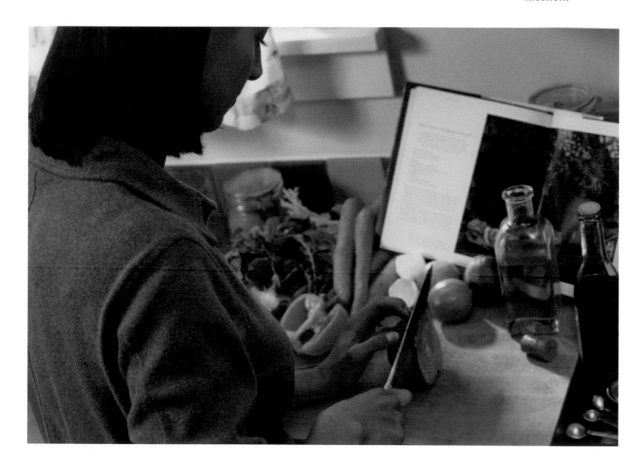

Utensils and cooking techniques

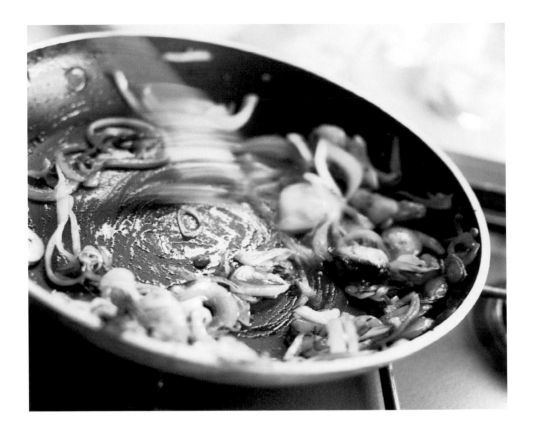

SHRED/ BEAT

Sometimes, to make purees, pastes, creams, or soups, we need to crush the ingredients to fuse them together and form a product with variable consistency and flow. There are several tools at our disposal, such as potato masher, mortar, or hand blender (such as "pimer") or blender (such as "turmix"). There is also a wide range of electric grinders, some with multiple functions, such as those known as food processors.

The mortar requires greater effort and time, but it is good for grinding food in small quantities. It needs to be as heavy as possible (stone or marble) so that it will not move while using. Metal mortars are more suitable for health food stores and pharmacies, where they work with dry goods. Those made out of wood absorb juices, which leads to harmful bacteria.

The traditional potato masher is good for making purees or softer dough, but it is being replaced by electric mixers these last few decades. You can prepare a cream or soup by boiling mashed vegetables and then dissolving them in the broth used for cooking by whisking by hand and mixing with oil. If you do not have enough time, crush the ingredients with the electric mixer.

Thermomix semiprofessional devices work not only for soups and creams, but also for a variety of hot and cold dishes and recipes. They are expensive, but their usefulness is indisputable.

Mixers let you do many things in the kitchen (sauces, whipping cream and egg whites, etc.). Table grinders, similar to those for coffee, let you shred all kinds of spices and cheese. Although they can still be found, they are being replaced by electric grinders.

There are countless tools to facilitate cooking, from a garlic press to seed and grain grinders, which are very popular in Germany. However, common sense and practice should help you choose what is best for you. Remember that having more kitchen utensils does not make you a better cook.

GRIND

You can find all kinds of quality whole grains, especially in health food stores but for those who prefer to buy organic grains in bulk and grind them at home slowly, there are grinders (electric or hand cranked). Some even allow you to make your own grain flakes. Grinders can be a little pricey, so shop around.

COOKING FOOD

Most foods we eat have been peeled, cut, crushed, ground, and heated with fire. Even though raw diets exist, certain foods (potatoes, soybeans, some varieties of beans, eggs, etc.) require cooking since they contain certain toxic substances that are destroyed by heat.

- **Boiling.** This is one of the most universal cooking methods: immerse food in boiling water. Keep in mind two things: always use the right amount of water and allow for a certain cooking time. By boiling food, they release minerals, trace elements, and other nutrients that make cooking broth. Should you cover the pot? Prevent any of these elements from disappearing with the heat is convenient by covering it, although inevitably certain ingredients are lost or transformed by boiling.

Boiling makes grain easier to digest and is very good for preparing foods such as legumes, vegetables, pasta, and eggs.

The broth can be taken with boiled or stored food, but eat it as soon as possible to avoid losing its nutritional properties through oxidation.

- **Steaming.** It is one of the healthier cooking techniques and more advisable than boiling. Prevents losing a lot of minerals and trace elements.

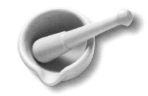

You can crush small amounts of food with a stone or marble mortar.

The secret of a good cut: the knife

Stainless steel knives have taken over the market, but there are still some made out of ordinary steel, sometimes more for nostalgic memory than anything else. Although they can be sharpened better, this type of knife tends to oxidize and darken quickly, so it is not recommended for use. But if you have one at home and you want to keep it, then clean it, dry it thoroughly, and smear it with oil.

Get a whetstone (fine-grained sandstone) to have your knives always ready. If it has a very jagged edge or the tip of the blade is broken, then dispense with the knife and buy another one.

• **Stews.** It is great for preparing dishes in which food is to be consumed with broth. The preparation is identical to that of boiling, although it usually incorporate some oil and seasoning.

• **Fried and breaded foods.** Oil, when heated, alters the state of the oil's fatty acid chains and creates toxic substances that cause disorders over time. Keep it from getting too hot or start to smoke, and cannot be reused. The best oils for frying are olive and, secondly, sunflower and soybean.

Using batters are worse than frying, because the coating absorbs more fat. Foods like this are only recommended in winter or when making an effort that requires a lot of energy.

• **Grilled.** It is one of the best alternatives to fried foods, because it requires little oil and food retains all its nutrients.

• **Oven roasted.** Along with boiling and steaming, it is one of the most recommended cooking techniques. By cooking at medium temperature and for a long time, food will roast evenly and hardly lose any nutrients. Smear a little oil without dampening (this would only make food more fried than grilled)

• **Roasting on the grill.** It is one of the oldest cooking methods. Currently, it can only be done with barbecues, rustic fireplaces, or ovens. Before placing foods on the grill, take care that they do not flare up and burn immediately.

Overcooking almost completely destroys vitamin C and a good amount of B vitamins.

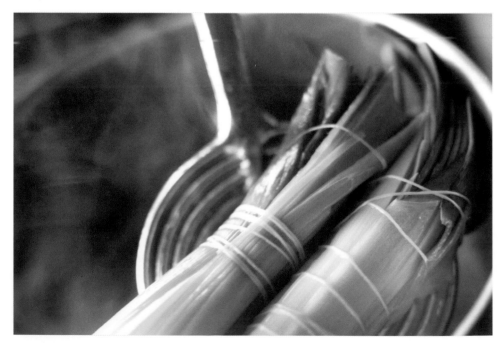

Cooking utensils

Cooking techniques have hardly changed, but ourhealth concernsregarding life and longevity is facilitating a series of improvements in cooking and meal preparation. For example, findings that make cooking with steam easier in modern kitchens: we are able to know, with precision of hundredths of a degree, at what temperature a steamed vegetable is cooking.

In this section we will take a brief look at tools and materials for cooking. We have already seen that it is best to use earthenware but there are other types of materials:

• **Fortified glass** utensils. They are convenient and their only disadvantage is that they let light in, resulting in some vitamin loss.

• **Stainless steel** is good as long as we use non-abrasive cleaning products (chlorine), or scouring pads that could scratch them and leave tiny bits of loose metal. If you do have to use these products to clean your stainless steel cookware, afterward, put a little vinegar with rhubarb root in the pot and bring to a boil to clear any remaining metal dust.

• **Cast iron** tools are much more acceptable and they are once again being distributed in Europe. Also those made with iron covered in **vitrified ceramic**. No bright colors should be chosen, as they may contain cadmium (harmful) in the glaze. Stop using them once they chip, because you risk contamination by iron oxide and they also destroy vitamin C.

• Regarding non-stick frying **pans** (with *teflon* coating), its safety is doubtful, since the coated layer is made of a substance that lets off poisonous fumes when it becomes very hot. The process for obtaining such a coating was surrounded by controversy because of its carcinogenic potential, which has not been sufficiently explained to consumers. In addition, the manufacturer has opted for a dubious solution: change the formulation slightly and most importantly change the name of the coating (with brands like "Silverstone" and others).

These pans can be good for cooking if soon after buying them you rub them with oil and warm them slightly to seal pores to the fullest. And then take extra care when cleaning (very gently with a soft sponge).

Practical tips

• Food should not be **overcooked**, otherwise they lose much of their nutritional properties.

• Although cooking takes less time using high heat, it is best to cook food at **moderate temperature**.

• Do not **reheat** food because they lose their nutrients.

• Burnt or very roasted foods are potentially **carcinogenic**, especially if eaten regularly.

• Use stocks, which have a significant amount of nutrients.

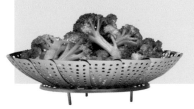

Utensils and cooking techniques

It is worth remembering from time to time the old saying: "The pan has a hole for hanging."

• **Pots.** Although conventional pots never disappear, there are new models for cooking in less time.

Thanks to their hermetic seal and exhaust valve, pressure cookers can increase the pressure and the water temperature inside (instead of boiling at 212° F (100° C), it does so at 230–248° F (110–120° C)), allowing foods to cook in almost half the time.

Controlled pressure cookers are similar to the above. They differ only in that their valve indicates the degree of pressure inside. But they allow you to more accurately control the temperature and cooking time, and are more expensive than conventional pressure cooker.

Thick-based pressure cookers prevent steam from getting out during cooking, so they require significantly less water or oil. Its bottom, which is much thicker than usual, allows heat to diffuse uniformly. Just as with controlled pressure cookers, their quality is unquestionable, but the price is high and worth thinking about before buying.

• **Stoves.** Gone are the old wood and coal stoves, which can only be found in some traditional restaurants. Today, everything is cooked with gas or electric stoves.

Suitable materials for cooking

• **Clay.** It is the best material for cooking. When choosing pots, we must ensure that they are unglazed because when heated they often give off small amounts of lead that can ultimately be very harmful. Clay goods are fragile, heavy, and bulky.However, they cook foods evenly and help retain their flavor and nutrients. You cannot put a clay pot directly over fire, as it would crack and break. To avoid this, heat it up gradually. If you are using a gas stove, place it on a diffuser plate.

• **Stainless steel.** This material is used for its strength and ease of cleaning (you have to wash it with soap and water, careful not to scratch the surface with the sponge). It is a good conductor of heat and cooks food evenly.

• **Cast or enameled iron.** Cast iron tools are coming back, which are an interesting alternative to the risk in using Teflon pans (when the coating starts to wear off). Enamel cookware is an alternative to stainless steel. If the enamel is in good condition, then it is an excellent material for cooking.

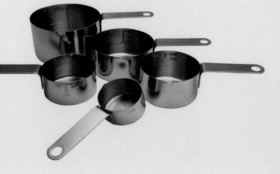

The first consume much more energy than the latter. Gas stoves burn butane, propane, or natural gas and leave significant residues. However, they require certain precautions, because if fire remains too high, then combustion gases can get mixed with food.

• **Ovens.** Electric and gas ovens have the same advantages and disadvantages as does the stove. Using the thermostat, clock, and speed controllers, we can roast different ways (heating from above, below, or both sides) and increase the range and characteristics of the dishes that can be cooked.

We already discussed the drawbacks of microwave ovens, so we won't dwell on it, but remember that they are not recommended.

• **The wok.** This simple traditional Chinese cooking utensil is for frying, sautéing, or steaming (with a steamer basket).The wok "paella" (actually it's not exactly a paella) is a cooking secret that comes to us from the East using crisp and colorful vegetables, or very aromatic rice . . . actually almost everything can be cooked using a wok. Choose a traditional wok made of iron or steel, of about a foot (35–40 cm) in diameter, with lid and cleaning brush. For cooking, it is better to use it with a gas flame.

• **Heat resistant glass.** Widely used for cooking in microwave ovens, their quality is comparable to that of stainless steel.

• **Wood.** Because of its low conductivity it is typically used for kitchen spoons. Wooden tools require some care: they cannot be washed with soap and need to be waterproofed with oil frequently so they do not get ruined.

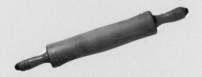

• **Aluminum.** It is not recommended because heat, salt, and food acids corrode it and make it dissolve in food.

• **Copper.** Although it is alloyed with tin, it tends to dissolve, so do not use it.

• **Teflon.** It is good for non-stick pans, so it is often used to coat all types of plates and pans. Its use should be monitored, however, because if the layer peels off, it becomes very harmful. So its use is not recommended, unless it is brand new.

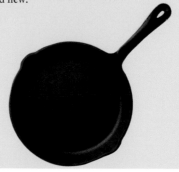

Utensils and cooking techniques

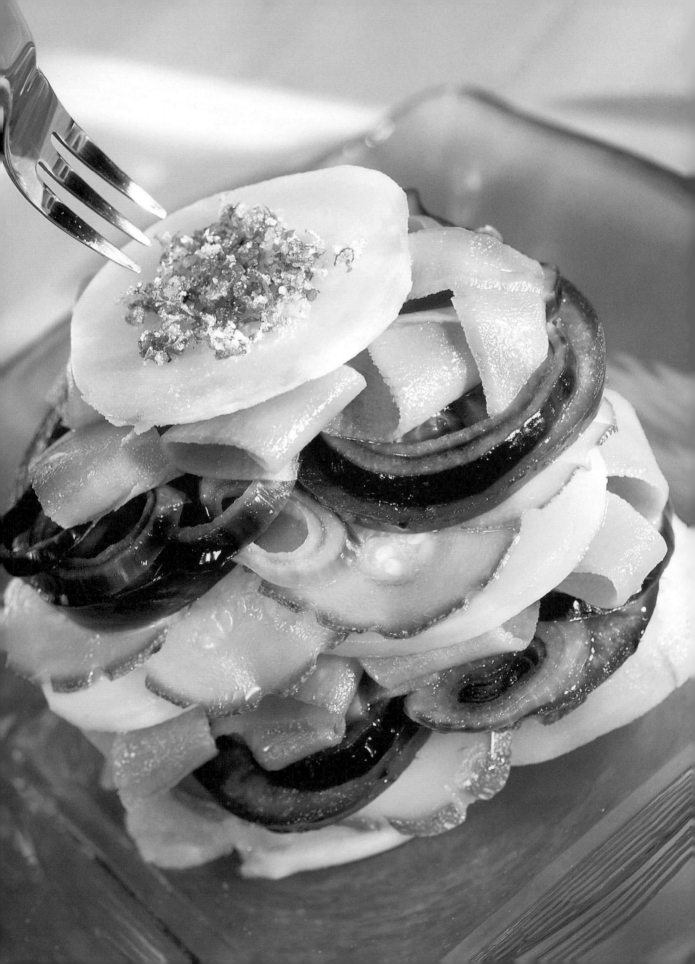

Recipes

6 Assorted salads

Vegetable broth: A medicinal food

Hot and cold soups

Rice

Potatoes

Pasta

Vegetables

Pizzas and quiches

Crêpes and potato patties

Oriental dishes

Mushrooms and special dishes

Desserts

Juices and drinks

Guide to eating well when you are short
   on time

The best and worst diets

Glossary

All greens salad

Ingredients
(serves 4)
- 4 artichokes
- 1 garlic clove
- Extra virgin olive oil
- 1 organically grown lemon
- Chives
- Sea salt
- 4 tender cabbage leaves
- 12 baby spinach leaves
- 1 red chicory bud (radicchio)
- 1 watercress bunch

Remove the outer leaves of the artichokes and trim the ends, leaving only the bottom part. Halve the artichokes and use a teaspoon to remove the fuzzy center, if any. In a mortar, crush the garlic and make a sauce by adding the oil, lemon juice, finely chopped chives, and salt. Cut the artichokes into thin slices and let them marinate in this sauce, while preparing the remaining ingredients. Use cabbage leaves as edible bowls and fill them with spinach, radicchio that was cut into strips, along with chives cut into quarters lengthwise, artichoke slices, and watercress. Season with the same sauce and garnish with thin strips of lemon peel.

Couscous salad

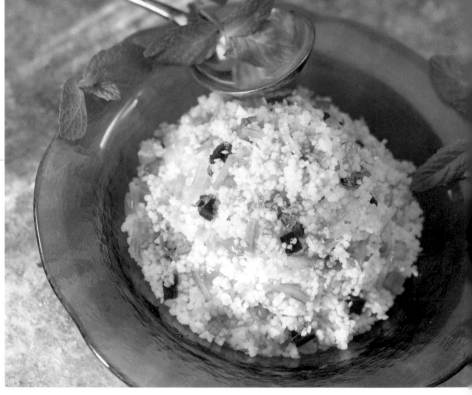

Ingredients
(serves 4)
- 3 cups (500 g) couscous
- 4 cups (1 l) of water
- Juice of 2 oranges
- 6 tomatoes
- 2 green onions
- 2 carrots
- 2 celery stalks
- 1 red or green pepper
- 8 lettuce leaves
- 2 garlic cloves
- 2 sprigs of parsley
- 2 sprigs of fresh mint
- Olive oil, tamari, yeast, and sesame for seasoning

Soak the couscous in water and orange juice for half an hour. Add two grated tomatoes. Peel and chop the onions and put them in water. Grate the carrots and chop the celery, bell pepper, tomato, and lettuce. Mince the garlic, parsley, and mint. Add all to the couscous and season to taste. It is best to first toast and crush sesame with a little sea salt, turning it into gomasio.

Red cabbage salad

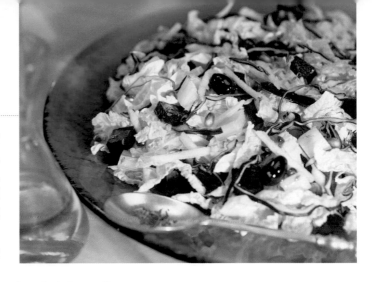

Wash both cabbages, remove the hard center and cut them into strips. Rinse off the beets, peel and dice. Clean and dice the celery. Peel and grate the apple. Make a colorful salad combining both heads of cabbage and adding the olives.

For the dressing, crush cumin in a mortar then add oil and soy sauce.

Mix well and pour over salad. Top with pomegranate seeds and serve with sliced lemon on side.

Ingredients (serves 4)

- 1/4 white cabbage
- 1/4 red cabbage
- 1 cooked beet
- 2 celery stalks
- 1 apple
- 20 black olives
- 1 teaspoon (5 g) cumin
- 4 tablespoon (6 cl) olive oil
- 4 teaspoons (2 cl) soy sauce
- 1 pomegranate
- 1 lemon

Corn and pomegranate salad

Cut the radishes in the shape of flowers and leave in ice water mixed with vinegar, until they open up. Cut the endive or lettuce into small pieces. Sprinkle the corn kernels and pomegranate seeds on top. Garnish with radish flowers and grated carrot. For the dressing, crush the garlic and pistachios in a mortar, and add oil to make a paste. Add herbs, lemon juice, and tamari. Mix and pour over the salad.

Ingredients (serves 4)

- 6 radishes
- 1 curly endive or lettuce
- 1/2 cup (100 g) sweet corn kernels
- 1 pomegranate
- 1 carrot or beet

For the dressing:

- 1 garlic clove
- 10 shelled pistachios
- 2 1/2 tablespoons (4 cl) olive oil
- 1 pinch of herbs
- 1 teaspoon (5 ml) lemon juice
- 4 teaspoons (2 cl) tamari

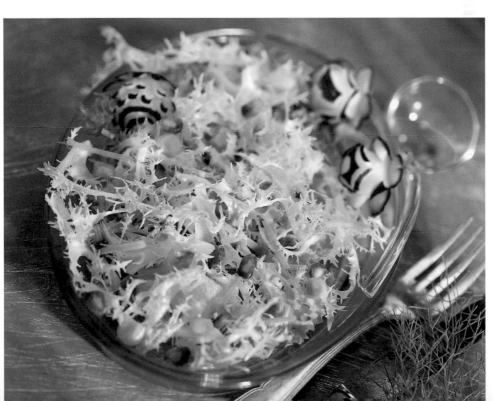

String salad

**Ingredients
(serves 4)**
- 4 white cabbage leaves
- 4 red cabbage leaves
- 4 carrots
- 2 raw beets
- 2 green apples, peeled
- 3 ounces (80 g) assorted sprouts (fenugreek, watercress, alfalfa)

This salad is notable for its julienned vegetables (cut into very thin strips). To make them, roll together white and red cabbage leaves and cut very thinly. Grate the carrots, beets, and apple with the thickest part of the grater. Add the sprouts, mix the ingredients well, and place in a bowl. A few tablespoons of green mayonnaise (see page 148) go great with this salad.

Tip: Serve this salad in a clear bowl to make it more attractive and appetizing.

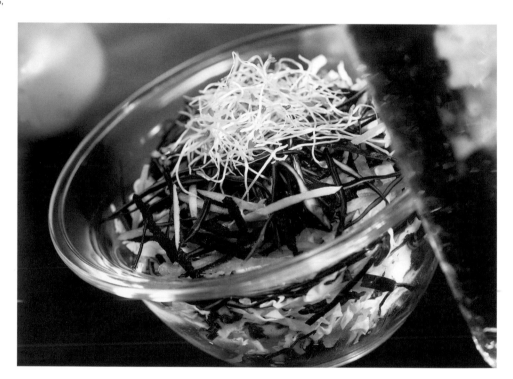

Mexican salad

**Ingredients
(serves 4)**
- 1 head of lettuce
- 1 tomato
- 1 ripe avocado
- Some corn kernels
- Fresh cilantro
- Oil and salt
- Some corn chips

Wash and cut lettuce, place a few leaves at the bottom of a wide bowl, then add remaining lettuce and the tomato slices (peeled and seeded) mixed with avocado slices. Then add corn kernels and cilantro leaves. Dress with oil and salt, and serve with corn chips.

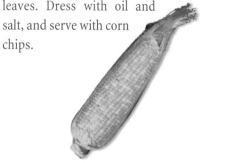

Rice salad with crispy broccoli

Begin by toasting the rice dry, stirring constantly. When you begin to smell its nutty aroma, pour all of the water into the pan, cover, and let simmer until all water is absorbed.

While it cools, prepare the remaining ingredients: slice garlic cloves and mix with the pepper and a bit of olive oil in a skillet over low heat for about three or four minutes. Then remove from pan and set aside. Turn up the heat and fry the broccoli in the same oil. After about five minutes turn off the heat. Cut the carrot into ribbons using a peeler and in a bowl mix the rice, broccoli, carrots, garlic slices, and pumpkin seeds. Make a salad dressing using tamari and a trickle of olive oil.

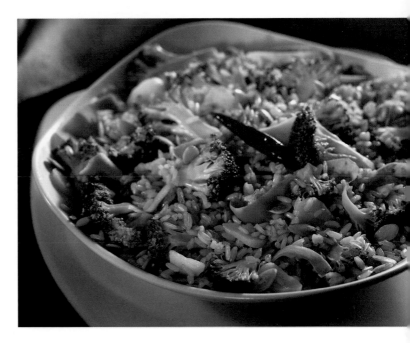

Ingredients (serves 4)
- 4 1/4 cup (1 kg) brown rice
- 8 cups (2 l) of water
- Olive oil
- 2 garlic cloves
- 1 chili pepper
- I broccoli
- 1 carrot
- 1/4 cup (20 g) pumpkin seeds
- Extra virgin olive oil
- Tamari

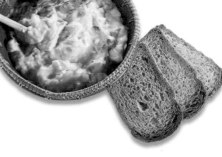

Vegetable crudités with guacamole

Cut the avocado in half and remove the pit. Scoop out the flesh into a bowl and reserve. Dice the onion and tomato into small cubes. Next, mash the avocado with the lemon juice, chopped cilantro, tomatoes, garlic, and onion. Then add the salt and chili powder to season.

Ingredients (serves 4)
For the guacamole:
- 3 ripe avocados
- 1/2 onion
- 3 tablespoons freshly squeezed lemon juice
- 2 tomatoes, peeled and seeded
- 1 garlic clove
- 1 pinch of salt
- 1 tablespoon (5 g) chopped fresh cilantro
- 1 pinch of chili powder

For the crudité:
Fresh seasonal vegetables (celery, peppers, carrots, cauliflower, cucumbers) cut into strips

Sautéed vegetable couscous

Ingredients (serves 4)
- 1 cup (1/4 kg) couscous
- Salt
- Extra virgin olive oil
- 1/2 cup (100 g) green beans
- 12 dried apricots
- 1 cup (200 g) cooked chickpeas
- 1 green onion
- 3 garlic cloves
- Parsley

Couscous

Place the couscous in a bowl with salt. Boil water with a tablespoon of olive oil. Add the couscous until it covers about a third of an inch (1 cm) of the saucepan. Simmer until water is absorbed.

Vegetables

Wash, cook, and drain the green beans. Cut each dried apricot into 4 pieces and cut the pepper into short, thin strips. Wash and drain the chickpeas. In hot oil, fry the onion, garlic, green beans, chickpeas, and peppers. Mix all ingredients, garnish with chopped parsley, and serve.

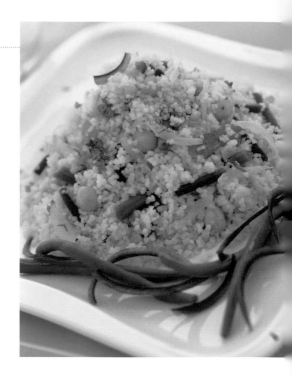

Sautéed vegetables

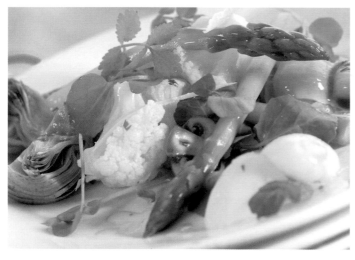

Chop the artichoke into quarters, cut the cauliflower into small florets, and discard the hard stalks of the asparagus.

Steam the vegetables and set aside.

Boil the potatoes without too much water then mash them with the potato masher, adding some of their cooking liquid as needed. Season with salt, pepper, and olive oil. For a stronger flavor, use oil marinated with garlic.

Clean the mushrooms and sauté in a pan with the vegetables.

Serve on a bed of watercress and mashed potatoes. Add the vegetables and sprinkle with Parmesan and parsley. Season with garlic oil.

Ingredients (serves 4)
- 2 artichokes
- 1/2 cauliflower
- 1 bunch green asparagus
- 3 potatoes
- 8 (200 g) mushrooms
- 5 cups (150 g) watercress
- 1 cup (100 g) Parmesan cheese
- Extra virgin olive oil
- Parsley
- Salt
- Pepper

Fruit salad in green tea syrup

Syrup

Cut a third of an inch (1 cm) of ginger root. Peel, grate, and set aside.

Make the green tea, add 5 tablespoons brown sugar, and bring to boil. Let it simmer for about 10 minutes.

A minute before removing from heat, add a pinch of cinnamon and ginger juice that you get from squeezing the grated ginger.

Fruit salad

Peel and cut the fruit into even chunks. Place them in clear cups and cover with the syrup. Keep it in the refrigerator until serving.

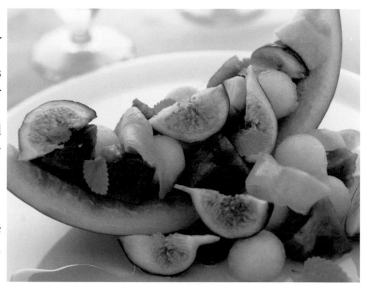

Ingredients (serves 4)
- Ginger root
- 1/2 cup (350 ml) green tea
- Brown sugar
- Cinnamon
- 1 3/4 cup (1/4 kg) watermelon
- 1 3/4 cup (1/4 kg) honeydew melon
- 1/2 lb. (1/4 kg) figs
- 1 extra-large (1/4 kg) peach

Avocado salad

Slice the tomato into wedges and cut the onion into very thin strips (use only as much as you like).

Soak the chili in warm oil until it acquires a spicy flavor.

Mix the cilantro in a mortar with olive oil and add salt to taste.

Slice the avocado and arrange on a plate with tomatoes and onion. Top with bean sprouts. Season with cilantro oil and a few drops of chili oil.

Ingredients
- 1 tomato
- Onion
- Chili
- Olive oil
- Cilantro
- Sea salt
- 1 avocado
- Bean sprouts

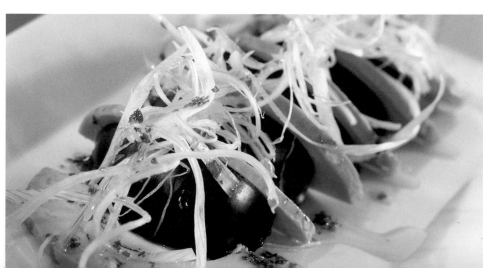

Catalan grilled vegetables

Ingredients
(serves 4)
- 6 potatoes
- 8 ripe tomatoes
- 4 onions
- 4 eggplants
- 2 ripe peppers
- 2 garlic cloves
- Extra virgin olive oil
- Salt
- Pepper

Wash unpeeled vegetables.

Make an incision around the potatoes and at the top of each tomato. Cut the onions crosswise and prick eggplants with a fork.

Preheat oven to 400° F (200° C), with heat at the top and bottom, and broil the potatoes, tomatoes, onions, eggplants, and peppers on a baking tray lined with foil.

Flip the vegetables every 10 minutes.

After 30 minutes, remove the tomatoes, peppers, and eggplants. Leave onions and potatoes 15 more minutes.

Allow vegetables to cool a little. Then, peel them and cut into long strips.

Season with garlic, oil, salt, and pepper.

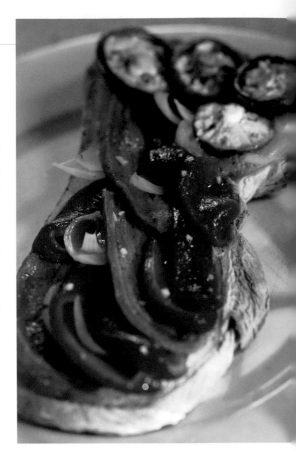

Fusilli pasta salad

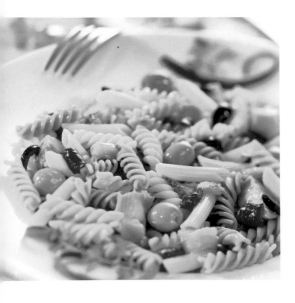

Ingredients
(serves 4)
- 1 eggplant
- 2 red peppers
- 2 cups (1/4 kg) rotini
- 2 cups (1/4 kg) penne
- 1/2 cup (100 g) artichoke hearts
- 10 green olives, pitted
- 10 black olives, pitted
- Capers
- Extra virgin olive oil
- Apple cider vinegar

Bake the eggplant and grill the peppers. When cool enough to handle, peel, remove seeds, and cut into chunks.

Boil the pasta in plenty of salted water and a little oil until it is al dente. Drain and season with two tablespoons of olive oil.

Cut artichokes into quarters. Add artichokes, eggplant, peppers, both types of olives, and capers to the pasta. Mix them all together. Season with plenty of oil and a tablespoon of apple cider vinegar. Mix and let cool.

Very green salad

Remove the outer leaves of the artichokes and trim the tips, leaving only the base. Halve them and remove the fuzzy center.

Make a sauce by crushing the garlic and adding oil, finely cut chives, lemon juice, and salt.

Cut the artichokes into thin slices and marinate in the previous sauce for about half an hour.

Use cabbage leaves as edible containers for the spinach, chopped chives, radicchio strips, watercress, and sliced artichokes.

Add a dressing made with the same sauce and serve immediately.

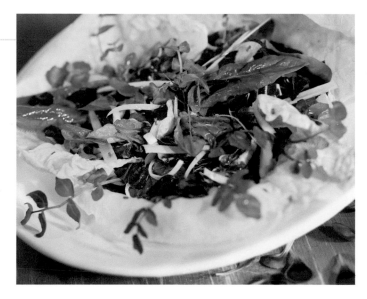

Ingredients (serves 4)
- 4 artichokes
- 1 garlic clove
- Extra virgin olive oil
- 1 chive
- 1 lemon
- Salt
- 4 cabbage leaves
- 12 spinach leaves
- 1 radicchio
- 1 watercress bunch

Mixed lettuce with marinated tofu

Dice the tofu and place in a bowl. Add oil and soy sauce. Cover the bowl and leave to marinate for an hour.

Wash the lettuce and cut it into large pieces.

Grill the marinated tofu. Cook for about three minutes until crisp.

Serve lettuce with the tofu and bean sprouts.

Ingredients (serves 4)
- 12 ounces (350 g) tofu
- 1 cup (1/4 liter) extra virgin olive oil
- 1 teaspoon (1/2 cl) soy sauce
- 17 ounces (1/2 kg) mixed lettuce
- 3 ounces (100 g) bean sprouts

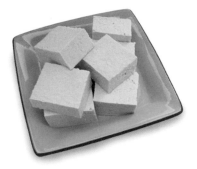

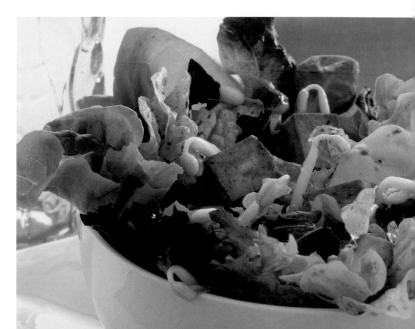

Recipes

Vegetable broth: A medicinal food

The nutritional and healing properties in vegetable broth make it one of the few cooked foods that are natural medicine. It can be had anytime: during an illness or in case of a fever, and even while fasting.

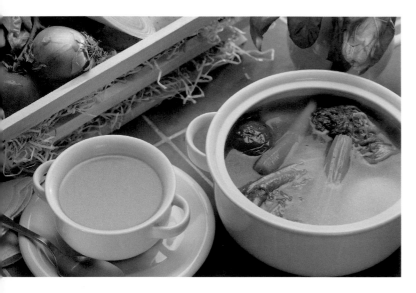

Ingredients
- Celery, carrots, onions, turnips, lettuce, endive, tomato, and garlic
- Extra virgin olive oil
- Salt

MILD VEGETABLE SOUP

It is ideal for healthy people and for those suffering from health problems, such as flu or liver disease. It is also recommended as first solid foods for infants, as well as a base for soups and porridges. In short, anyone can eat it.

It also allows variations to suit certain palates, by simply adding or substituting ingredients.

Vegetable broth recipe could not be simpler: boiling vegetables in water. Choose them well, chop them, put them in a pot, and cover with water.

BASIC RECIPE

There are many vegetables that we can use to prepare our broths. Each has certain healing properties and mix extremely well. All vegetables are boiled together for an hour and strained.

Cook at low heat. Meaning that after it first boils, only a few bubbles should surface.

The aromas and flavors of the vegetables will emerge after boiling. The broth should simmer over low heat, covered, to have a more concentrated flavor.

After the broth has simmered for about 45–60 minutes, drain out the vegetables.

Leftovers should stay uncovered until they are cold. Then cover and store in the refrigerator. You will have it ready any time to make soup.

HOW TO FLAVOR BROTHS

For extra flavor, add a splash of olive oil and herbs: thyme, marjoram, bay leaf, parsley, etc.

If it tastes too sweet, do not necessarily add more salt; it is better to give it a slight spicy or acidic flavor using pepper, pressed garlic, or lemon juice. A few drops of tamari (soy sauce) also enhance the flavor of the broth.

If you are fasting or have a fever, forget about using salt and oil.

Variations

The following broths are simple variations of basic broth. They are particularly good for illness or during fasting, but they are also great any time.

Diabetic's broth

This recipe is a real pleasure that anyone can enjoy. It is made with the same ingredients, but substitute rice for soybeans or rolled oats. Boil for one hour (10 minutes in a pressure cooker).

The diabetic's broth uses very little salt, and should not contain sugar, dry legumes, rice, bread, or spices.

Vegetable broth for fasting

We used to think that fasting was just about drinking water, but fasting can include vegetable broth, as more and more experts recommend. However, it is best to practice fasting under medical supervision, particularly if it is done over a long period of time.

This is one of the recipes:
Ingredients
- 4 cups (1 l) of water
- 1 lb (1/2 kg) carrots
- 1/2 leek
- Some celery and a little parsley

Boil all ingredients for 10 to 20 minutes. Drain and season with a pinch of sea salt and yeast. For more intense flavor, add dill, basil, or parsley.

Broth for transitioning to a meatless diet

For those who want to gradually eliminate meat from their diet we suggest a particularly dense vegetable broth that is tastier and more nutritious than the basic vegetable broth.

It is made with the same ingredients as above, but you add lentils, peeled peas, and lightly fried tomato, onion, and garlic. Drain the vegetables and blend them for a tasty vegetable puree.

It is very nutritious, but it takes more to digest than simple vegetable broth, so it is not suitable for people with health problems or a weak stomach.

Soups and purees

Making changes in the basic recipe can give you more flavorful results: you can cut the vegetables thinly and eat them in the broth. Once the broth is done cooking, you can blend it and the vegetables together. And if you drain out the broth and add grits or oatmeal or other grains you get a soup.

Practical tips

• Broths help you get the most out of hard or dry parts of vegetables that cannot be used in salads.
• Make sure the vegetables are organically grown (without pesticides) and do not let them soak too long before cooking, or you risk losing some of their vitamins and minerals.
• Do not throw anything away! When buying vegetables, we are used to throwing out "waste" (outer leaves of the cabbage, leaves of turnips and carrots, green part of leeks . . .) that contain an abundance of chlorophyll.
• Minerals are concentrated in the darker green leaves, so do not throw them out. The leaves and stalks of turnips, carrots, and radishes are delicious and are full of these nutrients.
• Let your intuition be your guide. Depending on the ingredients you use, certain flavor will predominate. The combinations are infinite.

Gazpacho

Ingredients
(serves 4)
For the gazpacho:
- 2 red bell peppers
- 8 ounces (250 g) ripe tomatoes
- 1 cucumber
- 1 onion
- 3 garlic cloves
- 3.5 ounces (100 g) bread crumbs
- 4 cups (1 l) of water
- 4 tablespoons (6 cl) vinegar
- 5 1/2 tablespoons (8 cl) olive oil
- Salt

For garlic croutons:
- 6 slices white bread
- 4 tablespoons (6 cl) of extra virgin olive oil
- 1 crushed garlic clove

Wash, peel, and remove the seeds from the vegetables. Then place all the ingredients in a blender and puree until smooth. Let cool in the fridge while preparing the croutons and garlic.

Preheat the oven to 350° F (180° C). Remove the bread's crust and cut it into one-third of an inch wide (1 cm) cubes. Crush the garlic and mix it with the oil. Drizzle the bread cubes with the oil and garlic mixture, and bake for ten to fifteen minutes, turning them until golden on both sides.

Serve gazpacho cold, with a bowl of garlic croutons. Alternatively, serve with diced onion, pepper, and cucumber.

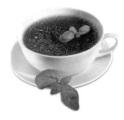

Tip: Add chopped shrimp to the gazpacho for a delicious and refreshing dish.

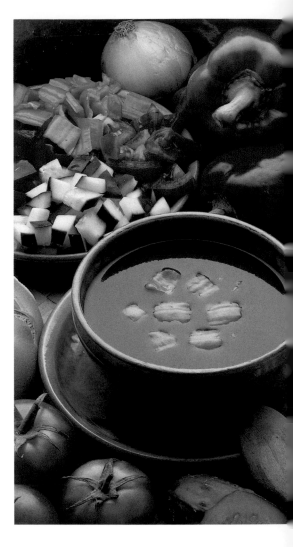

Onion soup

Ingredients
(serves 4)
- 3 3/4 cup (2 kg) onions
- Butter
- 6 cups (1 1/2 l) vegetable broth
- Oregano
- Grated Swiss cheese

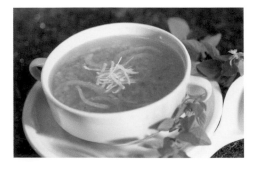

Peel and crush the onions and brown them in a little butter over low heat.

Add the vegetable broth and a pinch of oregano. Season to taste.

Serve with grated Swiss cheese.

Vichyssoise

Melt the butter in a skillet and fry the onions over low heat (peeled and sliced) until tender, but without browning them.

Then peel and dice the potatoes. Remove the green part of leeks, clean, and slice.

Boil six cups (a liter and a half) of salted water and add the potatoes, leeks, and fried onions. Cook for twenty minutes.

Blend with an immersion blender until creamy. Add the heavy cream, stir well, and let cool in the refrigerator. Serve cold.

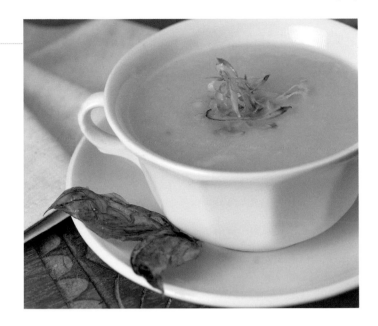

Ingredients (serves 4)
- 3/4 stick (75 g) butter
- 2 bunches (250 g) onions
- 10 ounces (300 g) potatoes
- 4 (600 g) leeks
- 4 cups (1 l) of water
- Salt
- 1/2 cup (150 g) heavy cream

Cream of zucchini

Peel and cut the zucchini, potatoes, and cauliflower. Then boil with herbs in four cups (a liter) of salted water for forty minutes.

Strain the vegetables (keeping the liquid) and puree them, adding the reserved cooking liquid as needed to obtain a creamy consistency.

Cut the whole wheat bread into cubes and fry in abundant oil.

Bring the pureed vegetables to a boil, remove from heat, and add the heavy cream.

Serve hot with the bread.

Ingredients (serves 4)
- 3 zucchini
- 2 large potatoes
- 1 cauliflower
- Nutmeg, pepper, salt, and bay leaf
- 2 cups (1/2 l) of water
- 4 slices whole wheat bread
- 1/2 cup (150 g) heavy cream

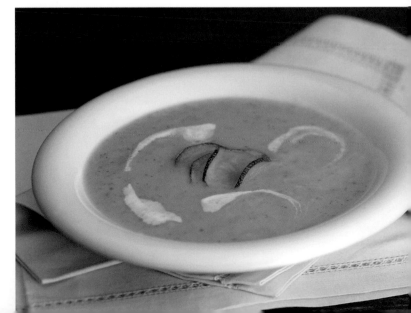

Curry rice

Ingredients
(serves 4)
- 1 cup (200 g) brown rice
- Salt
- 3 onions, chopped in large pieces
- 2 garlic cloves, minced
- 4 tbsp. olive oil
- 1 red pepper, chopped
- 1/2 cup (100 g) peas
- 1 teaspoon curry
- 1/2 cup (100 g) Emmental cheese

Cook the rice in salted water.

Meanwhile, in another pan fry the onion and garlic in 4 tablespoons (6 cl) oil and add the chopped pepper and peas. Fry the ingredients and simmer for about five minutes.

When most of the water has absorbed, mix the rice, onion, curry, grated cheese, and a little salt if needed. Mix the ingredients well, stirring with a spatula.

Finally, cover the pan and leave to simmer until all the water is absorbed and rice is tender.

Place the rice on a platter and serve hot.

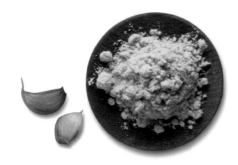

Rice casserole

Ingredients
(serves 4)
- 1 1/2 cup (300 g) brown rice
- 4 tablespoons (6 cl) olive oil
- 2 diced onions
- 1/2 red pepper, chopped
- 1 garlic clove
- 1 (500 g) Swiss chard
- Fresh ginger
- Salt
- 1 handful of currants
- 1 handful of toasted hazelnuts
- Bay leaf and thyme
- 1 parsley bunch

Cook the rice. Meanwhile, heat the oil in a large saucepan. Once hot, fry the onion until brown, add the red pepper, and minced garlic.

Then add the chard, clean and cut into small pieces. Stir and cover the pan so that it cooks in its own juice.

Once the chard has softened, add the rice (along with the remaining liquid), a tablespoon of ginger juice (grate a little and squeeze it with your hand), salt, currants, hazelnuts, bay leaf, thyme, and chopped parsley.

Stir a little and let simmer covered until all water has evaporated.

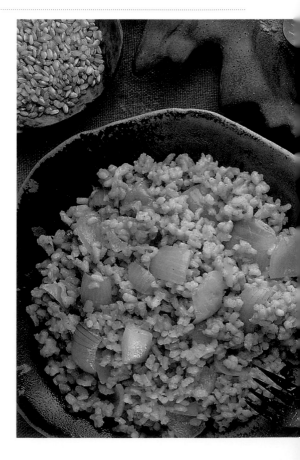

Indian rice

Cook the rice and meanwhile, heat the oil in a large saucepan. Once hot, fry the onion until tender. Add the carrots and stir from time to time; if it seems like it is about to burn, add a little water.

Set aside half a glass of water that the rice was cooked in and use it to dissolve the curry with a little salt, powdered cinnamon, and a teaspoon of ginger juice (grate a little and squeeze it with your hand). Then add the onion and carrot to the rice (along with the water that still remains), along with the water in which the spices were dissolved, as well as the apple slices.

Mix well, cover, and leave to simmer until all the water is absorbed.

As previously noted, it is important to let rice stand for about fifteen minutes.

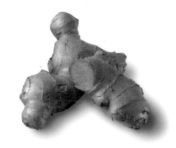

**Ingredients
(serves 4)**
- 1 1/2 cup (300 g) brown rice
- 4 tablespoons (6 cl) olive oil
- 3 chopped onions
- 2 sliced carrots
- 1 teaspoon (5 g) curry
- Salt
- 1 teaspoon (5 g) cinnamon
- Fresh ginger
- 2 golden apples

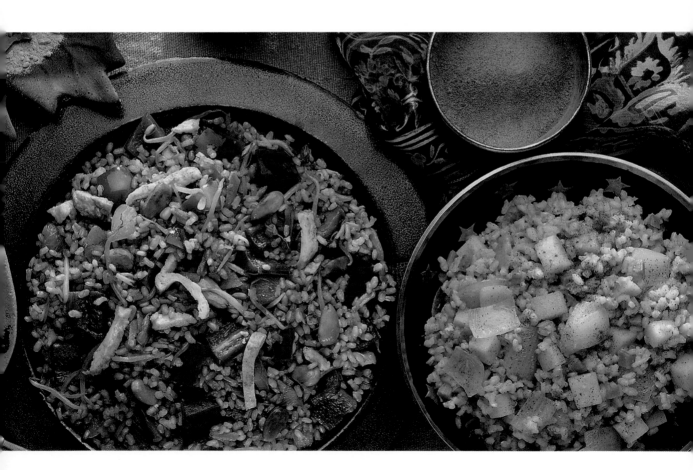

Rice with zucchini

Ingredients (serves 4)
- 4 1/4 cups (1 kg) brown rice
- Olive oil
- 8 cups water
- Sea salt
- 3 zucchini
- 1 onion
- 1 garlic clove
- 3.5 ounces (100 g) grated cheese
- 1 1/2 tablespoons (20 g) butter

Boil rice as follows: place oil in a large pan and fry the rice for one minute. Add 8 cups water and one teaspoon of salt. Bring to boil and let simmer forty minutes.

Wash and grate the zucchini without peeling; leave in a colander for half an hour. Next, peel and chop the onion and fry it with garlic in a pan. Add the drained zucchini and sauté everything for fifteen minutes over low heat. Mix rice with zucchini, sprinkle grated cheese, and butter.

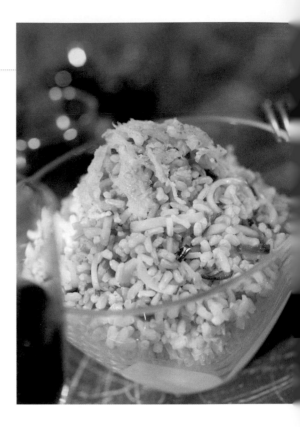

Thai rice

Ingredients (serves 4)
- 8 cups (2 l) of water
- 2 cups (400 g) basmati rice
- 2 garlic cloves
- 2 onions
- 1/2 carrot
- Olive oil
- 3 2/3 tbsp (60 g) soy sauce
- 1 teaspoon (5 g) Garam Masala, turmeric, or curry
- 1 teaspoon (5 g) brown sugar
- 1 teaspoon (5 g) chili powder

Place water and rice in a saucepan and bring to boil; cover the pan, bring the heat to low and cook until the water is absorbed.

While rice is cooking, sauté garlic, chopped onion, and carrot in 2½ tablespoons (4 cl) oil. In a bowl, mix the soy sauce, spices, sugar, and chili powder. Finally, add the rice and sauce to the vegetables. Place on a serving plate and garnish with chopped chives.

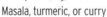

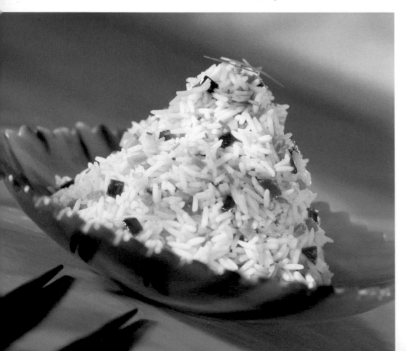

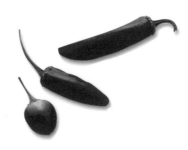

Vegetarian paella

Cook the rice and meanwhile, heat the oil in a large saucepan. Once hot, fry the onion until golden.

Add the remaining ingredients in this order: pepper, carrot, eggplant, zucchini (in the summer), artichokes, cauliflower (in winter), peas, green beans, and mushrooms. Every time a new ingredient is added, stir and cover the pan to soften it a little. If it is very dry and it could burn, add a little water.

Add soy sauce and herbs (amounts depending on taste).

Add the rice and, if needed, add a little water so it finishes cooking with the vegetables and is tastier.

Stir and taste (now is the time to add salt; later on it would ruin the consistency).

Cover the pan and cook over low heat until all the water (about fifteen minutes) is gone.

Place the garlic and the small bunch of parsley in a blender and mix with a little water. Then add it over the rice, without mixing.

Put the paella in the oven at 350° F (180° C) and leave until the water is absorbed. Once the paella is finished, let it stand fifteen minutes out of the oven with the lid on.

Tip: If you want to add color to rice, add some saffron.

Ingredients (serves 4)

- 5 1/4 cup (1 kg) brown rice
- 4 tablespoons (6 cl) oil
- 2 onions
- 1 red pepper
- 1 green pepper
- 2 carrots
- 1 eggplant
- 1 zucchini
- 4 artichokes
- 1 piece of cauliflower
- 1/2 cup (100 g) peas
- 1/2 cup (100 g) green beans
- 8 (200 g) mushrooms
- Soy sauce
- Pepper, oregano, thyme, basil, bay leaf
- Salt
- garlic
- parsley

Festive potato pie

**Ingredients
(serves 4)**
- 1 lb (1/2 kg) potatoes
- 1 carrot
- 1 onion
- 3 ounces (100 g) peas
- 2 eggs
- 9 ounces (300 g) mushrooms
- 1/2 stick (50 g) butter
- 3 tablespoons tomato sauce
- 1 can of red peppers, chopped
- 4 ounces (150 g) pitted green olives

Peel the potatoes, carrot, and half an onion, and boil together in salted water.

When they are cooked, drain water and mash them. Boil peas and set them aside.

Boil, peel, and slice eggs. Clean the mushrooms, cut them into small pieces, and brown them in the pan with the butter and chopped onion.

Mix the mushrooms with one egg, peas, tomato sauce, most of the chopped peppers, and chopped green olives. In a deep pan, well lined with baking paper, layer some mashed vegetables, then spread the filling, and cover with another layer of mashed vegetables.

Let stand one hour and unmold on a serving platter, garnish with the rest of the ingredients: the egg slices, olives, and chopped pepper.

Serve with salad, tomato sauce, or mayonnaise.

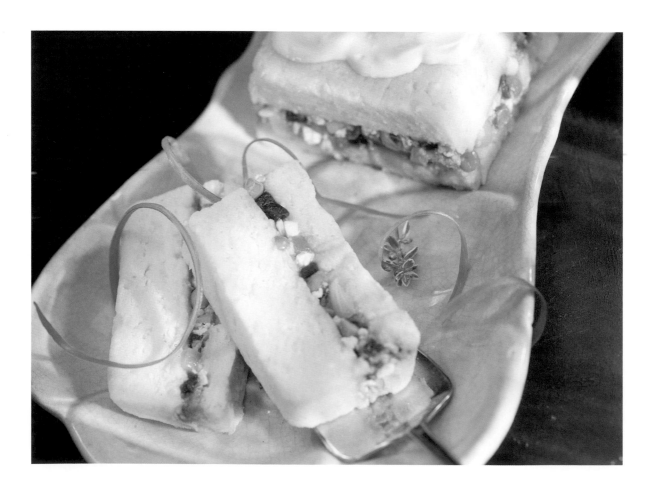

Couscous with raisins and chickpeas

Place the couscous in a fine colander and rinse under running water. Place couscous in steam cooker with a bit of salt, and cover with a cloth.

Fill the bottom of the steam cooker with hot water (halfway) and cook for five more minutes.

Meanwhile, rinse the raisins, remove the stems and dry them.

After the couscous has cooked for the first time, separate the grains with a fork, add the raisins and cook for five more minutes.

Mix the couscous again with a fork, add the butter in small portions. Add the drained chickpeas. Cook for five more minutes.

Serve in a deep dish.

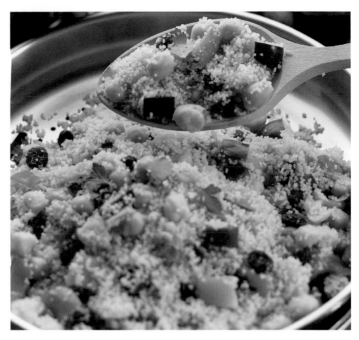

Ingredients (serves 4)
- 2 1/3 cups (400 g) couscous grains
- Salt
- 1.5 ounces (40 g) raisins
- 1 stick (100 g) butter
- 1 1/2 cups (300 g) cooked chickpeas

Chezal cup

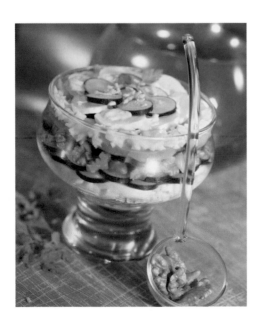

Boil the egg, peel and cut the cucumber, and slice the radishes. Rinse and dry the mushrooms and then slice them and sprinkle with lemon. Cut the chervil, walnuts (large pieces), and avocado (long slices, cut in half and sprinkled with lemon). For the sauce, mix the cayenne pepper with the remaining lemon, add cream, and season with pepper. Take out the egg yolk and chop the whites.

In a crystal goblet, place avocado, egg whites, mushrooms, radishes, walnuts, cucumber, and chervil. Cover in sauce and mix all ingredients.

Ingredients (serves 2)
- 1 egg
- 1/2 cucumber
- 1/2 bunch of radishes
- 5 ounces (150 g) mushrooms
- 1 tablespoon lemon juice
- 1 bunch of chervil
- 20 walnuts
- 1 avocado
- 1 pinch of cayenne pepper
- 2 1/2 tablespoons (4 cl) whipping cream
- Mixed pepper

Herbed gruyere-asparagus spirals

Ingredients
(serves 4)
- 1/4 stick (25 g) butter
- 1 ounce (25 g) grated Parmesan
- 6 ounces (175 g) cottage cheese
- 1/2 cup (150 g) heavy cream
- 4 egg yolks
- 4 egg whites, whipped
- 3 tablespoons chervil and parsley
- Sea salt and pepper
- 1 bunch (400 g) asparagus
- 7 ounces (200 g) grated gruyere

Preheat oven to 400° F (200° C).

Cover a long pan with parchment paper, smear it with butter, and sprinkle with grated Parmesan.

In a bowl mix ¼ cup (60 g) cottage cheese with heavy cream, egg yolks, and herbs. Season it and add the whipped egg whites. Pour into the mold, spread it, and bake for fifteen minutes. Unmold upside down on parchment paper. Place another piece of parchment paper on top, and flip right-side-up again for the next step.

Making the asparagus:

If raw, steam the asparagus five minutes; if they are canned, that is not necessary.

Soften the rest of the cottage cheese with two tablespoons of water and spread over the baked layer. Place the asparagus in a row and roll the whole thing like a jelly roll. Sprinkle the top with grated gruyere. Serve immediately in slices, or heat it wrapped in aluminum foil for another fifteen minutes.

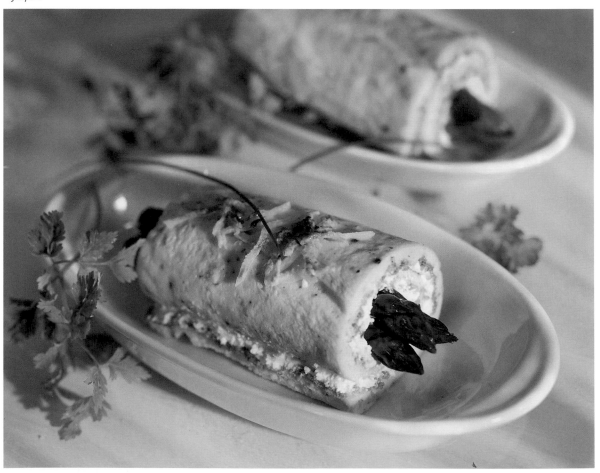

Delicate herb cake

Beat butter with sugar and add the eggs one by one. To the butter mixture, gradually incorporate the flour, then the yeast, to make a smooth and even dough. To this mixture, add the lemon zest, pine nuts, cheese, all herbs (minced), salt, and pepper. Mix everything and put in a deep and elongated mold. Bake for about one hour at 350F. Serve with tomato sauce.

Making the sauce:
Put olive oil in a pan and when hot, add the grated tomato. Add salt and, if needed, add sugar. When the sauce thickens, remove from heat.

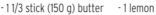

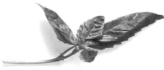

Ingredients (serves 4)

- 1 1/3 stick (150 g) butter
- 1/4 cup (40 g) sugar
- 6 eggs
- 2 1/3 cup (300 g) wheat flour
- 1 packet of powdered yeast
- 1 lemon
- 1/3 cup (50 g) pine nuts
- 3.5 ounces (100 g) grated Swiss cheese
- 1 parsley bunch
- 12 strips of chives
- Sprigs of fresh mint and basil
- Salt and pepper
- 3 (500 g) tomatoes, grated
- Olive oil

Stuffed squash au gratin

Halve the squash and remove the seeds. If the pulp is very thick, take out a little and bake with leeks. Steam both halves of the squash for five minutes; meanwhile, clean and cut the leeks into thin rings, and cut the rest of the squash into small pieces.

Boil both with a little water, until tender. Drain them, and in a bowl mix the beaten egg with the heavy cream. Season to taste using salt, pepper, and nutmeg, mixing well. Place this mixture inside the two squash halves and top off with cheese. Bake au gratin until golden brown.

Ingredients (serves 2)

- 1 small squash
- 1 bunch of leeks
- 1 egg
- 2 tablespoons heavy cream
- Sea salt
- Pepper
- Nutmeg
- 2 ounces (50 g) grated cheese

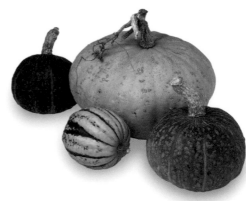

Pesto soup

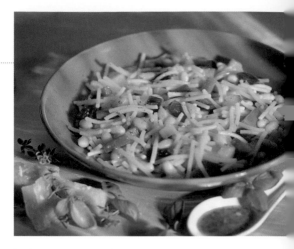

Ingredients
(serves 4)
- 3.5 ounces (100 g) cannellini beans
- 1 zucchini
- 2 1/4 cups (500 g) green beans
- 3 medium potatoes
- 2 tomatoes
- 1 bouquet garni: thyme, bay leaves, oregano, and winter savory
- 3 ounces (100 g) thick noodles

Soak the cannellini beans overnight; the following day, boil them for one hour. While boiling, clean the vegetables and dice them, and add the bouquet garni. Cook for twenty minutes, add the noodles, then cook for ten more minutes.

To make the sauce:
Chop the garlic and basil, add the pine nuts, and add the oil slowly with the salt. Thin out the pesto with a little broth before serving and add grated Parmesan.

Pesto sauce:
- 3 garlic cloves
- 1 ounce (20 g) fresh basil
- 1/3 cup (40 g) peeled pine nuts
- 1/3 cup (75 ml) olive oil
- Sea salt
- 1.5 ounce (40 g) grated Parmesan cheese

Green "mayonnaise"

Ingredients
- 2 1/4 cups (1/2 kg) green beans
- Juice of 1/2 lemon
- 1 teaspoon chopped parsley
- Sea salt

Cut the beans and cook over low heat in a covered pan with little water.

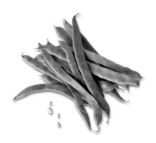

Once cooked, mix them in the blender with the lemon juice, parsley, salt, and a bit of cooking water (enough for a creamy consistency).

This sauce pairs well with rice salad.

Hot salsa

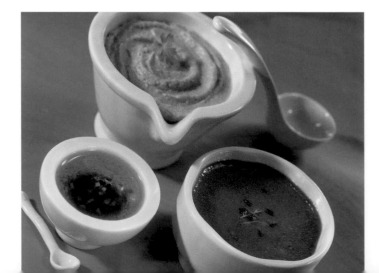

Place all ingredients in the blender and grind them. If the sauce is thick, add a little water for a smoother consistency.

Ingredients
- 3 tablespoons (5 cl) olive oil
- Sea salt
- 1/2 red pepper
- 1 tablespoon apple cider vinegar
- 1/2 chili
- 1 teaspoon roasted red Tabasco

Romesco sauce

Soak the peppers for a few hours or blanch them to be able to scrape the inner pulp.

Roast the garlic, tomatoes, and onions, and remove their skin and seeds. Mix chopped almonds, hazelnuts (roasted and peeled) and the remaining ingredients in a mortar or blender until well blended to create a paste. Peel the garlic, mince, and grind in a mortar along with the red pepper pulp (previously roasted or boiled). Add vinegar and enough oil into the mortar to create a sauce with the consistency of mayonnaise.

Use this sauce as a spread for toast.

Ingredients
- 2 spicy red peppers
- 2 garlic cloves
- 2 tomatoes
- 1 onion
- 1/3 cup (30 g) almonds
- 1/3 cup (30 g) hazelnuts
- 1 splash of apple vinegar
- Extra virgin olive oil
- Ground black pepper
- Salt

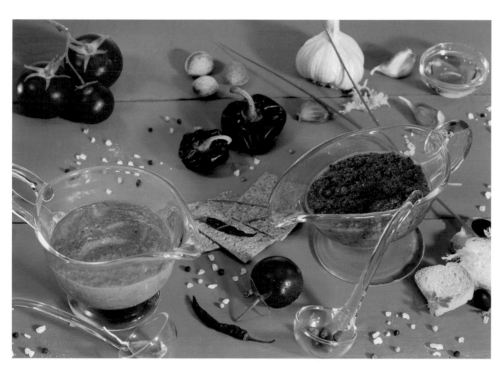

Cottage cheese and nuts

Peel and grate the apple. Then mix it with the lightly beaten cottage cheese, celery, and chopped walnuts and almonds. Add a teaspoon of honey, if desired, and serve for breakfast or as a mid-morning snack.

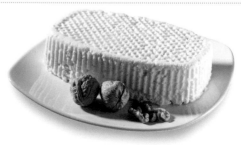

Ingredients
- 1 apple
- 3/4 cup (200 g) cottage cheese
- 1 sprig of celery greens, chopped
- 4 walnuts, chopped
- 4 almonds, chopped

Curry vegetable marinade

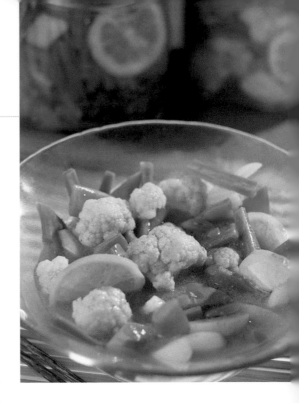

Ingredients
- 1 cauliflower
- 6 medium carrots
- 4 medium parsnips
- 1 celery
- 2 1/2 cups (500 g) green beans
- 2 lemons
- Sea salt

For the sauce:
- 2 tablespoons mustard
- 3 tablespoons curry powder
- Cayenne pepper
- 1 teaspoon ground ginger
- Ground cloves
- 1 small glass of vinegar or juice of 2 lemons
- 2 cups (1/2 l) oil

Prepare the vegetables the day before: cut the cauliflower into florets, peel the carrots and parsnips, and cut into julienne (in sticks). Clean and slice the celery (we will be using only the fleshy part of the stems). Clean the green beans and cut them into small pieces. Cut the lemons into thin slices.

Wash all vegetables and drain them, and place them in a bowl. Sprinkle them with a handful of sea salt and let marinate overnight in a cool place outside of the fridge.

The next day, steam them in the steam cooker with 4 cups (1 l) of water. Cover and steam the vegetables for three minutes, then uncover and cook for three more minutes.

Let the vegetables cool at least twenty minutes, drain them, and place in a salad bowl.

To make the sauce:

Mix together the mustard, curry, cayenne pepper, ginger, and cloves.

Add the vinegar (or lemon juice) and gradually add the oil, while whisking.

Season the vegetables with this sauce, mixing well. Fill the bowl with vegetables and before eating, leave them to marinate for a week in the refrigerator's fruit compartment.

Note: These vegetables keep well for up to three weeks in the refrigerator.

Tofu béchamel

Ingredients (serves 2)
- 1.75 ounce (50 g) tofu
- 4 cups (1 l) of water
- 1 teaspoon (5 g) paprika
- 1 teaspoon (5 g) soy sauce
- 4 teaspoons (2 cl) olive oil

Cut the tofu and boil it in a little water for about five minutes.

Then, using a blender, mix it with the rest of the ingredients.

This béchamel goes very well with vegetable pancakes.

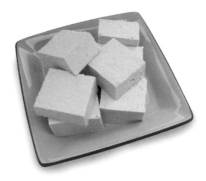

Fettuccine with tofu and broccoli

Dice the tofu and let it marinate a few hours in soy sauce, turning the cubes occasionally Boil the fettuccine in salted water and drain them.

Then roast the walnuts and steam the broccoli for about ten minutes.

Finely chop the onion, fry it with a little oil, and remove from heat.

Then do the same with the tofu.

Mix all ingredients and serve immediately.

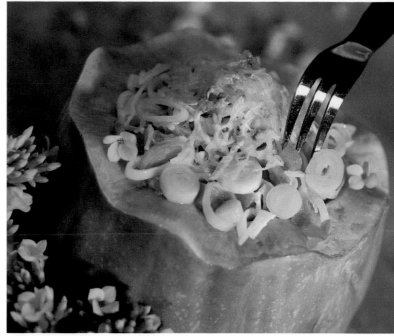

Ingredients (serves 4)
- 14 ounce (400 g) tofu
- 2 1/2 tablespoons (40 g) soy sauce
- 14 ounces (400 g) whole grain fettuccine
- 3.5 ounces (100 g) shelled walnuts
- 5 ounces (150 g) broccoli
- 1 onion
- 2 1/2 tablespoons (4 cl) oil
- Sea salt

Mediterranean lasagna

Prepare the seitan Bolognese sauce as follows: cook a little onion, celery, and carrot in a pan with butter (or organic margarine) over low heat.

Once browned, add the seitan, a little salt, pepper, nutmeg, and oregano.

Then add vegetable broth and a little tomato puree; boil for forty minutes, uncovered, and simmer, stirring frequently.

Slice the onion, eggplant, and zucchini, and fry them in a pan with olive oil for ten minutes, stirring occasionally. Meanwhile, cook the lasagna in salted water according to package directions (although some do not require cooking).

In a baking dish, place a layer of pasta on the bottom, then add a little seitan Bolognese sauce and finally add vegetables. Continue alternating layers of pasta, sauce, and vegetables.

Finish with a layer of pasta. Cover with the béchamel sauce and bake the lasagna over moderate heat, until brown.

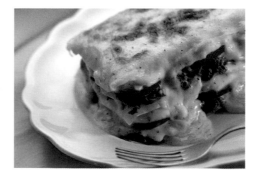

Ingredients (serves 4)
- 1 onion
- 1 eggplant
- 1 zucchini
- 4 tablespoons (6 cl) olive oil
- Whole grain lasagna
- Sea salt
- Seitan Bolognese sauce
- Béchamel sauce

For the sauce:
- 1 onion
- 1 celery
- 2 carrots
- Butter and seitan
- Salt, pepper, nutmeg, and oregano
- Vegetable broth
- Crushed tomato

Pizza

Ingredients:
- 2 1/2 tablespoons (25 g) of baker's yeast
- 3 tablespoons (5 cl) of warm milk
- 1 egg
- 4 teaspoons (2 cl) olive oil
- 2 1/3 cups (300 g) whole wheat flour
- 1 teaspoon (5 g) salt

Mix yeast in warm milk.

Beat the egg with olive oil and mix it with the milk and yeast, and then mix in the sifted flour with salt.

Work the dough with your hands for a few minutes and set aside covered in a warm place. Meanwhile, warm the oven and prepare the pizza toppings according to the chosen recipe or your own creation.

Stretch the dough by hand or with the help of a rolling pin or a clean bottle. The crust should be approximately 1/3-inch (one centimeter) thick.

Put it in a greased and floured pan, add the toppings, cover with a clean cotton cloth and let stand for ten minutes.

If the toppings look dry after ten minutes, sprinkle it with a little olive oil before placing in the oven.

Finally, put the pan in a hot oven for twenty minutes.

Pizza toppings:
The toppings should be cut into small pieces. First, spread a layer of tomato, then add the chosen ingredients (olives, pineapple, tuna, green and red pepper, corn, capers, carrots, etc.). Then cover with a layer of cheese.

It is important that the cheese used can melt; the most recommended cheese is mozzarella.

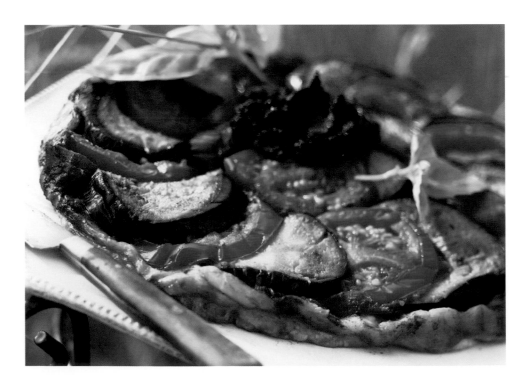

Dough for pies and quiches

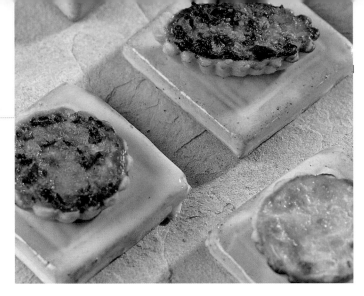

Mix flour, salt, and oil, and slowly add the water until forming dough that does not stick to the hands. Let dough stand while preparing the filling.

Tip: Make more dough by doubling or tripling the recipe. Divide it and put it in the freezer. So, next time there will be fresh dough readily available.

Ingredients

- 1 1/2 cup (200 g) fine wheat flour
- 4 teaspoons (2 cl) olive oil
- Warm water
- 1 teaspoon (5 g) sea salt

Cheese quiche

Cut the onion and sauté in 2 ½ tablespoons (4 cl) oil. Once softened, remove from the pan and let cool. Dice the tomatoes.

In a bowl, combine the cooked onions, diced tomatoes, eggs, herbs, salt, and pepper.

Line a pie dish with the dough from the quiche dough recipe, then fill the pie shell with the egg filling. Cook in the oven at moderate heat until the crust is cooked, 35 to 40 minutes approximately.

If you want a crispy crust, bake the dough first for a few minutes with a baking sheet underneath and then a few grains of dry legumes to prevent the dough from rising. Remove the paper and legumes, and fill as indicated above.

Bake it in the oven for about twenty more minutes. Alternatively, substitute shredded cheese with tofu.

Ingredients
(serves 4)
- 2 onions
- Olive oil
- 17.5 ounces (500 g) ricotta or cottage cheese
- 4 eggs
- Chopped fresh herbs
- Sea salt
- 3 tomatoes peeled and seeded

Leek quiche

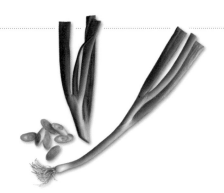

Select the white part of the leeks (we will keep the greens for a good broth) and steam them. Next, chop them and mix with the other ingredients, fill the quiche dough and bake.

Ingredients
(serves 4)
- 6 (1 kg) leeks
- 2 1/2 tablespoons (4 cl) oil
- 1 teaspoon (5 g) tarragon
- 2 eggs
- Sea salt

Recipes

Crêpes

Ingredients
- 3/4 cup (100 g) whole wheat flour
- 4 teaspoons (2 cl) olive oil
- 1 teaspoon (5 g) sea salt
- 1 pinch baking soda
- 13 tablespoons (5 cl) water

Place all ingredients in the mixer and beat until well blended. Let stand while preparing the filling.

To cook the crepes, put a few drops of oil in a medium or small nonstick skillet; put some of the batter in the pan (just under a ladle), and let it cook on one side. Then flip it over with a spatula to finish cooking on the other side. The thickness of the crepe will depend on the amount of batter used, so if the first one is a little too thick, use a little less for the following ones.

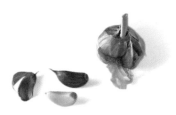

To make the filling:
Fill the crepes with ricotta, cottage cheese, or tofu; spinach with pine nuts and raisins; with tofu sautéed with onions and soy sauce; or mushrooms with garlic and parsley. It is best to use what we have at home or take advantage of seasonal food.

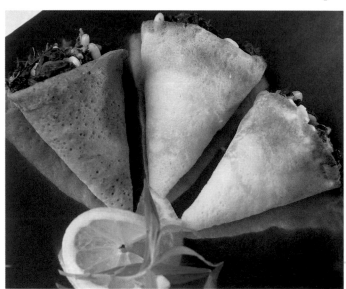

Potato patties

Ingredients
- 2 potatoes
- 2 Granny Smith apples, peeled and chopped
- 1/2 onion
- 1 egg
- 1/2 tablespoon whole wheat flour
- Nutmeg
- Sea salt
- Olive oil

Boil the unpeeled potatoes for five minutes; meanwhile, steam the apples in 4 tablespoons (6 cl) of water.

Next, peel and grate the potatoes and onions, and mix them with beaten egg, flour, and seasonings.

Using this mixture, make small patties and fry them on both sides. Make an applesauce from the cooked apples and let cool in the refrigerator.

Serve each diner a couple of hot patties with a generous spoonful of cool applesauce.

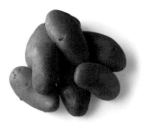

Maki sushi

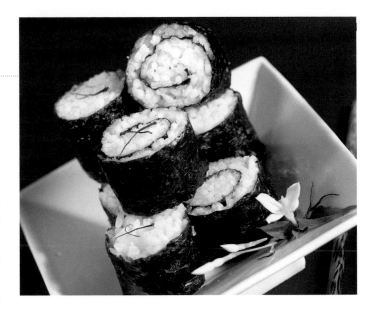

Lightly fry the onion in 2 ½ tablespoons (4 cl) oil and when browned, add the rice and saffron.

Add broth or boiling water, cover, and let simmer. When the water is absorbed the rice is ready, but it is better to give broth a try. If it needs more time, add a little more hot water until it is done cooking. Meanwhile, place all the sushi ingredients in a bowl and mix them well.

When the rice is ready, add it to the bowl and mix well with the sauce. Then wait for it to cool enough so you can grab it with your hands.

Then place the seaweed on the mat with the smooth side up (seaweed has a smooth side and a rough side) and spread a layer of rice over it using your hands.

Keep a glass of warm water with a few drops of rice vinegar nearby to wet your fingers. This simple trick keeps the rice from sticking to your hands when making the rolls. Leave a margin to the sides—about half an inch (1.5 cm)—and on top of the seaweed sheet—about three-quarters of an inch (2 cm). Then place the filling on top of the rice (along the center).

Prepare the filling:

The maki sushi is the most well-known sushi roll. It is filled with a myriad of possible ingredients, such as strips of salmon or tuna, cucumber, preserved daikon, dried mushrooms (after soaking for half an hour), dried gourd or kampyo, preserved ginger, omelet, or sesame seeds. Use what you have at home: cucumber, avocado, lettuce, carrots, peppers, or make an omelet. Of course, everything must be cut lengthwise into thin strips. So for example, you could use a little chopped lettuce, then a few strips of pepper and avocado, and add a little tofu mayonnaise.

Roll the sushi:

Use the mat for rolling, but only in the beginning, applying some pressure. Then finish rolling, press the bamboo mat around one last time, and tuck in the rice to keep it from spilling out the edges. Repeat the process using another seaweed sheet and keep the rolls until serving time. Then, dip a sharp knife in water and cut the rolls into slices, starting at the center and moving outward.

Serve with a small bowl of soy sauce and chopsticks.

Ingredients
- 2 tablespoons (20 g) chopped onion
- Olive oil
- 1/2 cup (100 g) brown rice
- 3 saffron threads
- Hot water or broth (1.5 more than the amount of rice)
- 2 sheets nori seaweed

For sushi:
- 3 tablespoons (50 ml) rice vinegar
- 1 teaspoon (5 ml) of mirin (rice wine)
- 1.5 tablespoons (20 g) brown sugar
- 1 teaspoon (5 g) salt

Vol-au-vent broccoli with Roquefort

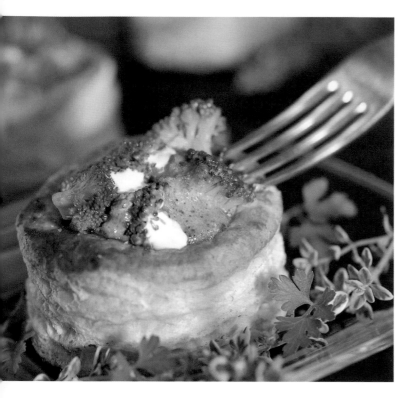

Soak the bread in water and then break it into small pieces. Grind together the garlic, parsley, olives and capers. Mix with beaten egg, heavy cream, and oil.

Steam the broccoli florets, place them on the vol-au-vent (should be small circular pieces), and cover them with a spoonful of the mixture. Add Roquefort cheese on top and bake half an hour, until golden.

Ingredients (serves 4)

- 1 slice of bread
- 1 garlic clove
- 1 small parsley bunch
- 24 pitted black olives
- 4 1/2 tablespoons (40 g) capers
- 1 egg
- 3 tablespoons (5 cl) heavy cream
- 2 1/2 tablespoons (4 cl) olive oil
- 8 broccoli florets
- 8 vol-au-vent puff pastry shells
- 2.65 ounces (75 g) Roquefort cheese
- Sea salt
- Pepper

Gnocchi with tapenade

Ingredients (serves 4)

- 14 oz (400 g) short pasta (gnocchi or macaroni)
- 4 garlic cloves
- 14 teaspoons (2 cl) olive oil
- 6 ripe tomatoes, peeled, and seeded
- Sea salt
- Brown sugar
- 3 tbsp (40 g) black olive paste
- 1 1/4 tbsp (10 g) capers
- Parmesan cheese

Boil the pasta and meanwhile prepare the sauce: slice the garlic thinly and put in an oiled pan over very low heat. Cut the tomatoes into small pieces and add them. Add salt, a pinch of brown sugar, and cook with the pan covered for fifteen minutes. Add the olive paste and capers. Place the cooked pasta in a deep bowl and mix in the sauce. Serve with slices of Parmesan cheese.

To prepare the tapenade

Black olive paté
Using a mortar, mix olives, garlic, capers, olive oil, and lemon juice until you get a smooth paste. It can be prepared a few days in advance and stored in the refrigerator.

Ingredients
- 9 ounces (250 g) pitted black olives
- 2 garlic cloves
- 2 teaspoons capers
- 5 ½ tablespoons (8 cl) olive oil
- Juice of 1 lemon

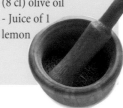

Spectacular Superfoods

Mushroom croquettes

Finely chop the onion and sauté with oil in large skillet; before they become golden, add mushrooms and continue sautéing.

Add flour and stir with a wooden spoon. Add cold milk, butter, and seasonings. Stir for fifteen or twenty minutes over medium heat until it thickens and does not stick to the sides of the pan. Let it cool off on a flat tray.

Roll out the mixture using the palms of your hand, cover in egg and bread crumbs, and fry in hot oil.

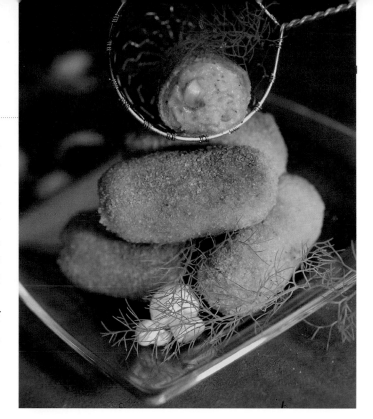

Ingredients

- 3 onions
- 9 ounces (300 g) mushrooms
- 1/3 cup (40 g) flour
- 1 1/4 cup (30 cl) milk
- 1/4 stick (30 g) butter
- Salt and pepper
- Nutmeg
- 1 egg
- Bread crumbs

Stuffed mushrooms

Separate the heads of the mushrooms from the stalks and rinse them in water with vinegar. If they are already very clean, simply wipe them with a damp tea towel.

Chop the stalks of the mushrooms as well as the shallots, garlic, and parsley. Fry them together in oil over low heat, until they begin to brown. Remove from heat.

Add the chopped seitan, bread crumbs soaked in a little milk and well drained, the egg, salt, pepper, and grated nutmeg. Mix well.

Fill the mushroom caps with the hash, pressing it in. Place them inside the steam cooker, on a bed of parsley.

Fill the lower compartment halfway with hot water and then add the mushrooms, cover the pot, and cook for fifteen minutes.

To serve, remove the stuffed mushrooms using a slotted spoon and place them in a bowl.

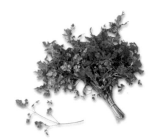

Ingredients

- 15 ounces (500 g) large mushrooms
- Vinegar
- 4 shallots
- 1 garlic clove
- 1 parsley bunch
- 4 tablespoons (6 cl) olive oil
- 8 ounces (250 g) chopped seitan
- 1.8 ounces (50 g) grated bread crumbs
- 1 cup (1/4 l) milk
- 1 egg
- Salt
- Pepper
- Nutmeg

Quinoa burger

Ingredients
- 1.75 oz (50 g) quinoa
- 4 cups (1 l) of water
- 1 ounce (30 g) tofu
- 1/2 roasted pepper
- 0.9 ounce (20 g) chopped parsley
- 1/2 garlic clove
- Whole wheat flour
- Olive oil
- Sea salt

Boil the quinoa, then reduce to a simmer and cook for fifteen minutes. Meanwhile, blend the tofu, roasted pepper, parsley, and garlic using a blender. Combine cooked quinoa with tofu mixture and enough whole wheat flour to be able to make the burger patties (it will yield two large patties or four small patties). You can grill, bake, or fry the patties in a little olive oil.

Quinoa

Cultivated for over 5,000 years by indigenous cultures of South America, quinoa has an unusual amount of protein as well as a large number of essential amino acids. Besides being easy to prepare, it can be used for salads or pastries.

Soy burger

Ingredients
- 9 oz (250 g) textured soy protein
- 2 tbsp (20 g) chopped onion
- .75 ounce (20 g) chopped tofu
- 1 cup (200 g) cooked brown rice
- Sea salt
- Bread crumbs
- 2 1/2 tablespoons (4 cl) oil

Place soy protein in hot water to hydrate; meanwhile, quickly sauté the chopped onions in an oiled pan. When the soy protein has softened, put it in the blender along with tofu, rice, and salt to taste, then grind. Use the resulting paste to make the patties.

If the paste is still very dry, add a little water. You can grill, bake, or fry the patties. For frying, first cover them in bread crumbs.

Serve them with tofu slices, fried tempeh, or some French fries.

(Textured soy protein is dehydrated soy available in health food stores. In addition, there is a wide range of products made from soy products: pasta soup, granules, etc., to add into our daily diet.)

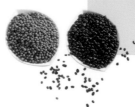

Soy

This is our number one food in our list of phytoestrogens because it contains isoflavones, which are substances that reduce hot flashes in menopause, inhibit the growth of cancer cells, help combat osteoporosis, and lower cholesterol. Alternatively, you can find isoflavone tablets, but there are so many ways to eat soy that you might as well try your hand at a recipe. You can meet your daily needs with a cup of soy milk or half a bowl of sprouts or tofu. According to the experts, Asian women are living proof of their many benefits because their health during and after menopause is significantly better than women in the West.

Marbled eggs

If you want to give hard-boiled eggs an original appearance, you can make them look marbled.

After piercing holes to keep the shells from cracking, cook them for ten minutes in a strong tea. Take them out of the tea and tap them to crack the shell without breaking it off.

Cook them for five more minutes to harden. Then chill them in water and peel off their shells for a pleasant surprise.

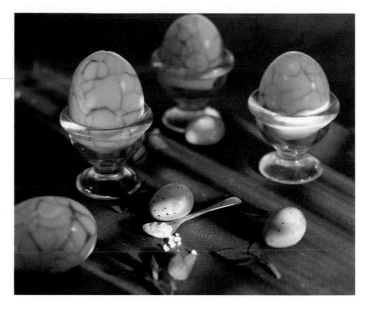

Cottage cheese balls

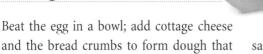

Beat the egg in a bowl; add cottage cheese and the bread crumbs to form dough that can be molded into ping-pong sized balls.

Boil the balls for five minutes in boiling water and in the meantime, grate the tomatoes then sauté with a little sea salt and oregano or basil.

Stir in the heavy cream to create a smooth sauce. Pour the sauce in a tray. Place the cheese balls in with the sauce and sprinkle with grated cheese. Finally, cook au gratin.

Ingredients
- 1 egg
- 1 1/3 cup (300 g) cottage cheese
- Bread crumbs
- 3 tomatoes
- Sea salt
- Oregano or basil
- 2 1/2 tablespoons (4 cl) heavy cream
- 2 ounces (50 g) grated cheese

Provençal omelet

Cut the leek and pepper into strips and fry in an oiled pan. Chop the tomato and add it to the pan with salt and tempeh.

To make the omelet, beat the eggs with a pinch of salt and pour half in a lightly oiled pan. When the egg begins solidifying, flip it to cook on the other side. Fill with vegetables, fold, and serve with a sauce.

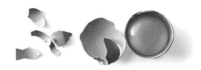

Ingredients
- 1/2 leek
- 1/2 green pepper
- 4 tablespoons (6 cl) olive oil
- 1 peeled and seeded tomato
- Salt
- 1 piece of sliced tempeh
- 3 eggs

Savory mushroom pudding

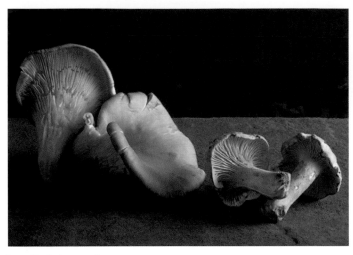

Wash and cut the mushrooms. Dice the carrot, onion, celery, leek, garlic, and tomato. Gently fry a fourth of the mushrooms and chopped vegetables in a little olive oil.

In a bowl, beat the eggs and add the cream, flour, remaining mushrooms (still raw), salt, and nutmeg.

Blend together both mixtures and use it to fill four molds brushed with margarine and sprinkled with bread crumbs.

Cook them in a double boiler at 275° F (140° C) for about thirty minutes.

Ingredients (serves 4)

- 2 lb (1 kg) mixed mushrooms
- 1 carrot, 1 leek, and 1 tomato
- 2 onions
- 1 small tender sprig of celery
- 2 garlic cloves
- Olive oil
- 4 eggs
- 4 cups (1l) of cream
- 2.5 tbsp (20 g) whole wheat flour
- Salt and grated nutmeg
- Margarine
- Bread crumbs

Round sandwich

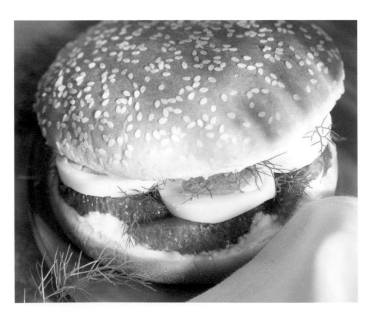

Slice the bun and take off some of the crumbs. In a bowl mix the mayonnaise, yogurt, and lemon juice, and spread this mixture over both pieces of bread. Insert the grapefruit wedges, sliced boiled egg, and fennel. Place the top slice to cover.

Ingredients

- 1 sesame bun
- 2 tablespoons mayonnaise
- 1 tablespoon yogurt
- Lemon juice
- 2 grapefruit wedges
- 1 sliced egg
- Some fennel stalks

Colorful pita

Dice the vegetables and fry in a little oil. Season with salt and curry. Once tender, warm up the pita to swell, open it, and fill it with vegetables.

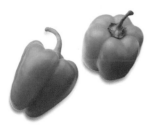

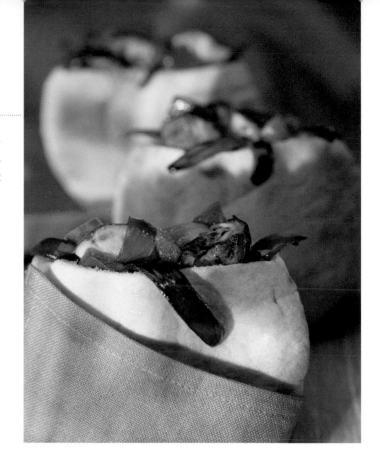

Ingredients

- 1/2 onion
- 1/4 eggplant
- 1 tomato
- 1/2 red pepper
- 1/4 zucchini
- Extra virgin olive oil
- Sea salt
- Curry
- 1 pita bread

Jasmine butter

Wrap a butter stick in cheese cloth, place it in a bowl full of jasmine flowers, and leave it overnight in a cool place to absorb the aroma. The next day, spread it on toast.

Jasmine has relaxing and invigorating properties. Small, very fragrant, and fresh, the white flowers are excellent for perfuming tea, fruits, sorbets, fruit salads, sweet creams, or with different fruits to prepare ice creams and jellies.

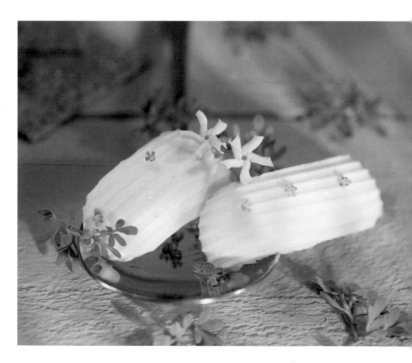

Ingredients

- 1 stick of butter
- 1 bowl of jasmine flowers

Little angels

Ingredients
(serves 4)
- 1 endive
- 1 beaten egg
- Flour
- Olive oil
- Honey

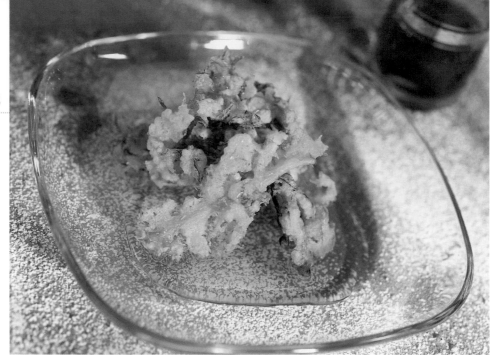

Remove the outermost leaves of the endive and wash thoroughly. Drain well.

Dip the leaves in beaten egg and flour. Once covered in batter, fry in plenty of hot olive oil, making sure not to burn them because of the large amount of water they contain.

Once fried and drained with paper towels, add honey to taste. Serve hot for dessert.

Spring rolls

Ingredients
- 1 ounce (20 g) cornmeal
- 4 teaspoons (2 cl) water
- 1 1/4 tablespoons (20 g) soy sauce
- 4 ounces (125 g) mushrooms, chopped
- 1 egg
- 2 1/2 tablespoons (4 cl) of sunflower oil
- 1 garlic clove
- .3 inch (1 cm) fresh ginger root, minced
- 3.17 oz (90 g) bean sprouts
- 1 green pepper
- 2.12 ounces (60 g) carrots
- 8 18 x 12 inch (45 x 30 cm) puff pastry sheets
- White pepper
- Salt

In a shallow bowl, mix the cornmeal with water, soy sauce, salt, and a little white pepper. Cover the mushrooms with this mixture and let stand for ten minutes. Beat the egg and pour in a small skillet to make a thin omelet. Let cool and cut into thin strips.

Place the wok over high heat until it gets very hot, add oil and fry the garlic and ginger, bean sprouts, peppers, and carrots for three minutes.

Remove and set aside. Remove the wok from heat, let cool and add the omelet strips and mushrooms.

Preheat oven to 400° F (200° C) and divide the filling into 32 parts. Stack all eight dough sheets one on top of the other, cut four strips of 4 x 12 inches (11 x 30 cm), and use a brush to smear oil on a strip of dough. Place some of the filling on one of the shorter ends of the dough, leaving .3 inch (1 cm) free on each side. Wrap the filling with the dough, fold inward and continue rolling until you reach the opposite end.

Bake the rolls, turning once, until golden, for fifteen or twenty minutes. Serve hot, with some soy sauce.

Potato soufflés with cheese

Bake the unpeeled potatoes in the oven for about twenty minutes. Before taking them out, check if they are cooked using a toothpick: if you can insert it into the center without a lot of effort, they are done.

Once cooked, halve them, peel them, and put them in a bowl. Mash them with a fork and let cool for five minutes.

Add the grated cheese and egg yolks, then add salt and pepper, mustard, and cayenne pepper.

In another bowl, beat the egg whites until stiff and add them gradually to the potato mixture. Mix well.

Fill the potato skins with this mixture, place on a baking sheet, and bake for fifteen minutes or until they turn golden brown. Sprinkle with chopped walnuts and serve immediately.

Suggestion:
• With tomato, cheese, olives, and parsley
• With tomato, corn, and hard boiled egg
• With cheese, pepper, and chives

**Ingredients
(serves 4)**
- 4 potatoes
- 5 oz (150 g) grated Cheddar cheese
- 3 eggs, separate the white from the yolk
- Salt and freshly ground black pepper
- 1 teaspoon (5 g) mustard
- Pinch of cayenne pepper
- Walnuts for garnish

Falafel

Puree the boiled chickpeas, season with a pinch of salt, pepper, and cumin. Add egg yolks, garlic, and chopped parsley. Mix well and take small portions to form little balls.

Fry in plenty of oil, and just before serving, sprinkle with the chopped parsley.

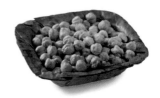

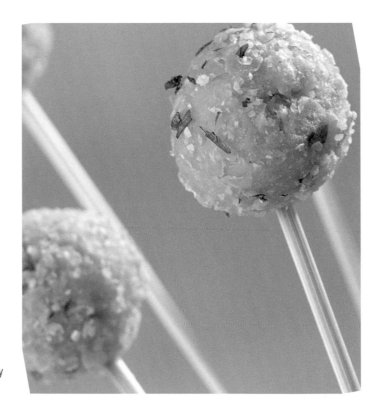

Ingredients
- 2 3/4 cups (500 g) cooked chickpeas
- Salt and pepper to taste
- 1 teaspoon (5 g) cumin
- 2 egg yolks
- 4 garlic cloves
- Chopped parsley
- Extra virgin olive oil

Banana cream

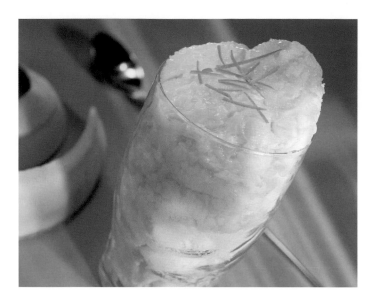

Peel and cut the fruit; drizzle the slices with lemon juice and put in the freezer until firm. Take them out and mix with honey using the food processor, pureeing until very smooth. Serve this ice cream in glasses sprinkled with orange zest.

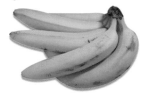

Ingredients
- 2 bananas
- 1 pear
- 4 teaspoons (2 cl) lemon juice
- 1 tablespoon honey
- Orange zest

Apple tarts

Ingredients
- 8 cups (2 l) of water
- 2 large apples
- 1/4 stick (30 g) butter
- 2 egg yolks and 1 whole egg
- 1/3 cup (70 g) brown sugar
- 6 1/2 tablespoons (10 cl) heavy cream
- Powdered cinnamon

Boil the water in the steam cooker and in the meantime, peel and core the apples, slice them thinly. Add the apples to four small heat-resistant ramekins that have been previously buttered.

Beat the egg yolks and whole egg with sugar, then add the heavy cream and continue beating a little more. Pour this cream into the ramekins over apples; cover the ramekins with kraft paper and steam for thirty minutes.

Remove and sprinkle each ramekin with cinnamon.

Cherimoya surprise

Ingredients
- 4 cherimoyas
- 2 oranges
- 2 ounces (50 g) grated coconut
- 2 tablespoons (40 g) liquid honey
- 2 walnuts
- 4 leaves of fresh mint

Cut the cherimoyas at the top and empty them out using a spoon. Halve the oranges and, before juicing, cut off a slice from each of the four parts. Mix the orange juice with the cherimoya pulp and strain using a chinois (mesh) sieve and a spatula to remove the seeds. Add the grated coconut and liquid honey and beat vigorously.

Serve chilled inside its own shell, supported at the base, with a slice of orange floating above, half a walnut, and a mint leaf. Drink with straw.

Peach and date chutney

Blanch peaches in boiling water, remove the skin and pits, and slice. Place all ingredients in a pan and heat slowly until sugar dissolves. When it starts boiling, cook over low heat for half an hour, stirring occasionally, until it thickens. Then let cool before using it to fill mason jars, which will be preserved for a month before serving.

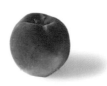

Ingredients
- 6 peaches
- 5 ounces (125 g) dates, pitted and sliced
- 3/4 cup (125 g) grapes
- 2 chopped onions
- 1 3/4 cup (350 g) brown sugar
- 2 garlic cloves, minced
- 0.71 oz (20 g) mustard seeds
- 1 oz (40 g) fresh ginger, chopped
- 6 shelled cardamom seeds
- 1 1/4 cup (30 cl) tarragon vinegar (or cider vinegar)
- 1 3/4 teaspoon (10 g) salt

Spring fruit salad

Remove the seeds from the cherries and apricots.

Dice the apricots and kumquats, and mix them together. Layer the fruits into 4 cups.

Dilute the almond cream by adding the juice of two oranges, and add finely chopped fresh mint.

Pour the cream into the four cups.

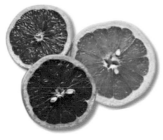

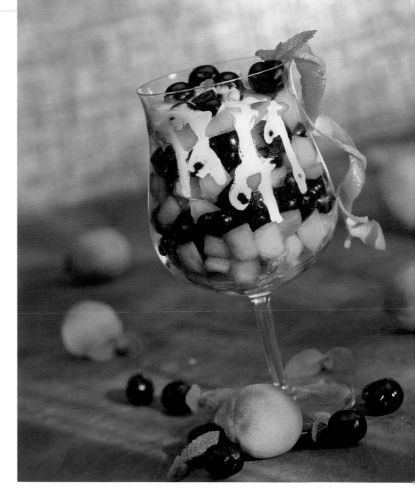

Ingredients
- 8 oz (250 g) kumquats
- 8 oz (250 g) apricots
- 8 oz (250 g) cherries
- 2 oranges
- 2 sprigs of fresh mint
- 4 tbsp (40 g) almond cream

Fruit salad and ice cream

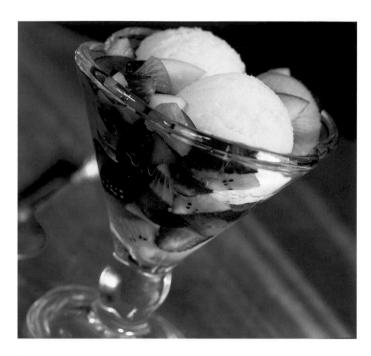

To make the ice cream, first mix the queso fresco, honey, and vanilla using a blender. Beat the egg whites until stiff, add them to the mixture, and put them in the freezer. Meanwhile, prepare the fruit salad by mixing sliced fruit with sugar and juices. Let cool. Finally, remove the ice cream from the freezer, stir well, and serve with the fruit salad.

Ingredients
For the ice cream:
- 7 oz (200 g) queso fresco
- 1 tablespoon (20 g) honey
- Natural vanilla
- 2 egg whites

For the fruit salad:
- 1/2 cup orange juice
- Juice of 1/2 lemon
- 7 oz (200 g) seasonal fruits
- 1 teaspoon (5 g) cane sugar

Lemon mousse

Ingredients
(serves 4)
- 4 cups (1 l) homemade lemonade
- 1 lemon
- .71 oz (20 g) agar-agar
- 3 tablespoons (60 g) honey
- 10.5 ounces (300 g) natural tofu
- Some strawberries or kiwis for garnish

Mix half a cup of lemonade with the agar-agar and stir until dissolved.

Then boil the rest of the lemonade, with sliced lemon, over low heat and stir constantly for ten minutes. Sweeten with honey, add dissolved agar-agar, and let cool slightly.

Put the mixture in a blender, grind and add the crumbled tofu slowly until soft. Serve in individual bowls and let cool in the refrigerator. Before serving, garnish with fresh fruit.

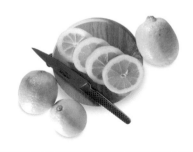

Little boats

Ingredients
- 4 cherimoyas
- 7 oz (200 g) blackberry jam
- 1/3 cup (50 g) blackberries
- 1.50 ounce (40 g) pollen

Start by cutting the cherimoyas lengthwise, hollow them out carefully so as not to damage the skins, and remove the seeds. Mix the pulp with jam and beat everything together.

Fill the half shells and garnish with some blackberries.

Sprinkle with pollen and serve cold.

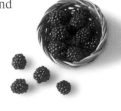

Cherry cake

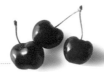

Wash and dry the cherries and remove their seeds. Beat butter with sugar and add the eggs one by one. Add sifted flour, together with the baking powder and salt. Mix it all together. Preheat oven to 350° F (180° C), ten minutes prior.

Butter an 8-inch (22 cm) round pie dish and pour in half of the batter. Layer all the cherries on top, then cover with the remaining batter. Bake until a toothpick comes out clean when inserted into the center of the cake.

**Ingredients
(serves 4)**
- 1.76 lb (800 g) cherries
- 1 1/2 tablespoon (20 g) butter
- 1 cup (200 g) sugar
- 4 eggs
- 2 1/3 cups (300 g) flour
- 1 teaspoon (5 g) baking powder
- 1 pinch of salt

Whole grain cookies

Grind the buckwheat flakes. Mix with sesame, chopped almonds, and baking soda. Mix warm butter and sugar with the rest of the ingredients. Finally add raisins and knead.

Let the dough cool a bit if it is too hard to work with. Heat the oven to 350° F (180° C) and prepare a greased baking sheet. Make small dough balls and flatten with a spoon. Place them on the baking sheet with some distance between them because they expand when baking. Bake for fifteen or twenty minutes.

Ingredients
- 1/2 cup (100 g) buckwheat flakes
- 1/3 cup (50 g) sesame
- 1 ounce (30 g) almond
- 1/4 tsp (1 g) baking soda
- 3/4 stick (80 g) butter
- 1.76 oz (50 g) cane sugar
- 1 ounce (25 g) raisins

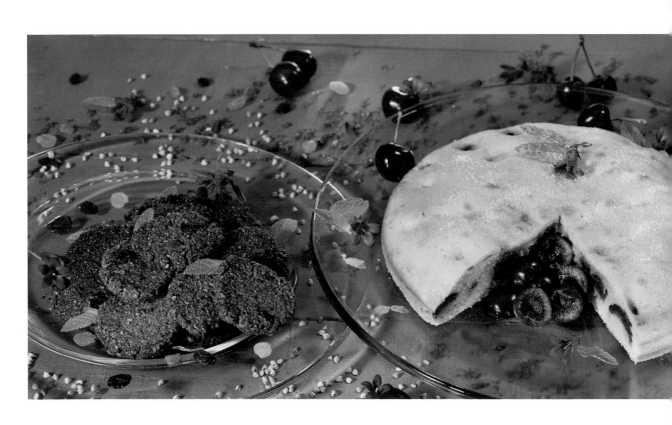

Saffron mousse

Ingredients (serves 4)
- 1 cup (200 g) whipping cream
- 1 1/4 cup (300 g) milk
- 15 saffron threads
- 4 eggs, separated
- 1/2 cup (120 g) sugar
- 1/3 cup (40 g) cornstarch
- 1.76 oz (50 g) agar-agar

Boil 1/2 cup (150 g) of whipping cream with the milk and saffron. Meanwhile, in a bowl, beat the yolks with the sugar until they're frothy.

Add cornstarch to the boiling cream mixture and stir, and then for a few minutes over low heat, stir constantly, until it thickens.

Meanwhile, cut the agar-agar in small chunks and, in a separate pot, cook with the rest of the whipping cream. Add the egg whites and proceed to carefully add the saffron cream, stirring just until the foam is even.

Garnish with saffron, grated orange, and grated chocolate.

Caramel pears

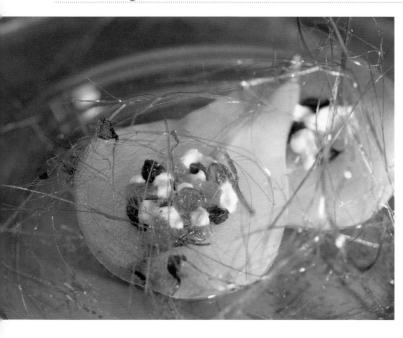

Peel, halve, and core the pears. In a heavy-bottomed pot caramelize the sugar slightly and add hot water to make some syrup. Add the pears and cinnamon stick and let simmer for ten minutes. Then place them on a serving tray with currants at the center. Mix the cream with the remaining syrup and pour it on the pears. Sprinkle with a little cinnamon.

Ingredients (serves 4)
- 8 pears
- 6 tablespoons (75 g) brown sugar
- 13 tablespoons (5 cl) water
- 1 cinnamon stick
- 1.76 oz (50 g) currants
- 13 tablespoons (5 cl) cream
- Powdered cinnamon

Sweet potatoes for dessert

Ingredients (serves 4)
- 2 sweet potatoes
- 4 peaches
- 1.41 oz (40 g) almonds

Bake the unpeeled sweet potatoes in the oven until they are very soft. Let them cool and then puree with peeled and sliced peaches. Pour the puree into individual containers and store in the fridge. Before serving, sprinkle with chopped almonds.

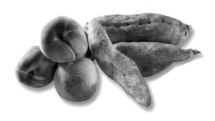

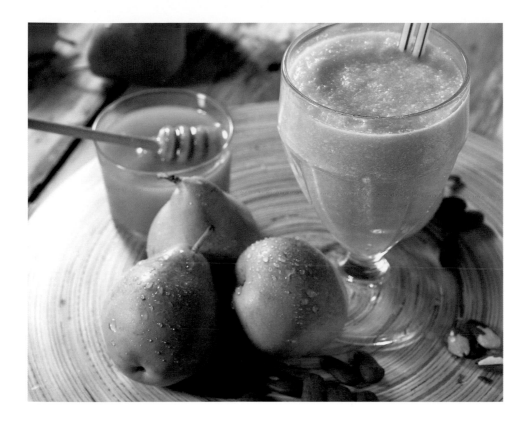

Almond and pear drink

First, blanch the almonds with boiling water and rub with a dry cloth to peel them well. Then, using a blender, grind the almonds, half the water, honey, and peeled and diced pears. Blend all ingredients until finely ground. Then add the remaining water and continue mixing.

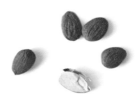

Ingredients
(serves 4)
- 4 cups (1 l) water
- 2 cups (200 g) almonds
- 3 tablespoons (80 g) raw honey
- 2 ripe pears

Sweet dates

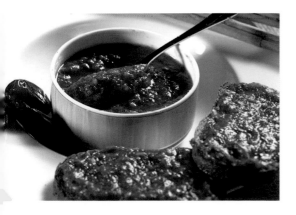

Bring the ingredients to a boil and cook over low heat until the dates are tender. Remove the cinnamon stick and grind until it has a creamy consistency.

Store it in the refrigerator, preferably in a glass jar. Serve as a side dish for cooked apples, breakfast cereals, or spread it on toast.

Ingredients
(serves 4)
- 1 cup (1/4 l) of water
- 10 ounces (250 g) pitted dates
- 1 cinnamon stick

Garnet granita

**Ingredients
(serves 4)**

- 7 oz (250 g) blueberries (or berries)
- 1/2 cooked beet
- 2 cups (1/2 l) red grape juice
- 1 cup (1/4 l) of water
- 1 1/4 tbsp (20 g) brown sugar
- 4 teaspoons (2 cl) lemon juice

Crush the fruit and beet, and set aside. Heat the grape juice, water, and sugar, and let it simmer for five minutes over low heat. Then mix the two and add the lemon juice. Let cool and place in a container for freezing. Take it out before it is completely frozen, and using a fork, scrape off any crystals that formed. Mix it slightly and serve in previously chilled glasses.

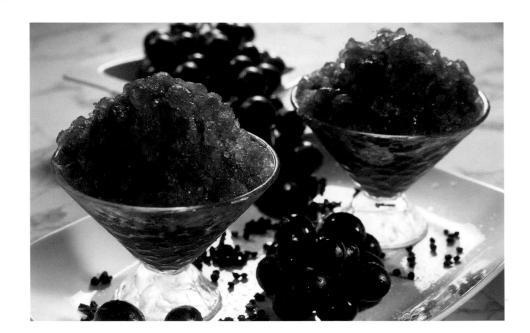

Green tea with spices

**Ingredients
(serves 2)**

- 1 ounce (40 g) green tea
- 1 orange peel and 1 lemon peel
- Nutmeg
- 2 vanilla pods
- Brown sugar
- Crushed ice (optional)
- Juice of 2 oranges
- Juice of 1 lemon

Place tea in the bottom of the pot and add the orange and lemon peels, a little nutmeg, and vanilla pod. Add brown sugar to taste and pour over boiling water. Cover to brew the tea and let cool.

To serve, add a little crushed ice, orange juice, and a few drops of lemon juice.

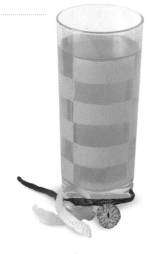

Juice with sprouts

Sprouts are one of the most wholesome new superfoods out there, and now it is easy to find them in health food stores or even prepare them at home. The most popular are soy and alfalfa (pictured), which is much easier to digest, whether sweet or spicy (mixed with germinated radish or mustard seeds). When preparing the juice, at the end simply add a handful of sprouts in a blender, but do not over do it because some sprouts have a strong flavor. Fresh onion and leek sprouts are also very good.

Tomato juice with sprouts is made the same way but using a blender.

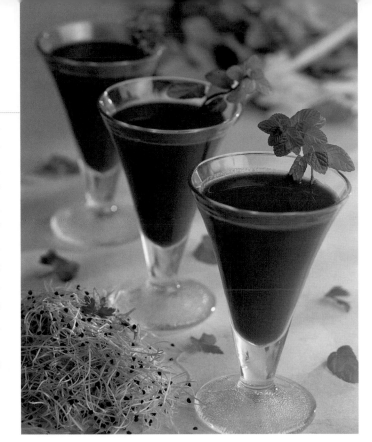

North-South smoothie

Wash the pears and apples, and cut them into quarters. Put pears, apples, and lemon in a blender and liquefy.

Add some strawberries and garnish with some edible flowers.

**Ingredients
(serves 2)**
- 2 pears
- 1 apple
- 1/4 lemon, peeled
- strawberries
- edible flowers (roses, chrysanthemums, etc.)

Orange cocktail

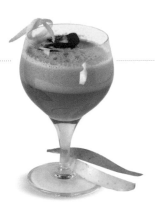

Peel the oranges and divide into quarters. Next, peel and chop the pineapple. Wash and de stem the grapes. Mix the fruit in a blender, and serve in glasses garnished with a slice of orange.

**Ingredients
(serves 2)**
- 2 oranges
- 2 thick pineapple slices
- 1 cup (200 g) red grapes

Guide to eating well when you are short on time

Many people think that eating healthy—with so little time outside of work—is almost an impossible task, and so eating sandwiches day after day solves everything. However, it is very important to find a solution, because our body "makes" energy, health, and disease. We need to make sure we are eating good food, no matter how little time we have.

It is not simply a matter of satiating our hunger just to keep working. We have to be aware that eating is one of the most important parts of the day. In fact, it is not that difficult planning nutritional meals.

All it takes is better organization, making good choices, and trying to have a balanced diet.

The following are some suggestions for having healthy meals at work:

PLANNING IS IMPORTANT
One of the first steps is trying to combine our personal tastes with our nutritional needs. In that sense, it is very useful to make a weekly schedule to try and vary our ingredients every day. Once this is done, we can go out and buy what we need for the week. This will keep us from eating the same things over and over again and from eating poorly.

It is very easy to create tasty and balanced dishes.

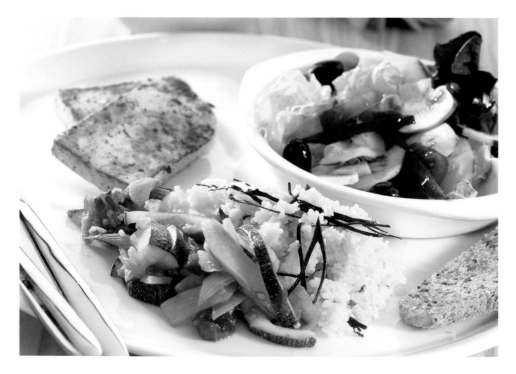

A Healthy Pantry

As we make the shopping list, we start to plan a diet for ourselves. Depending on what we buy, our food will be healthy and beneficial or harmful. You should have the following:

• **Legumes and whole grains:** better still if they are organic; if you have time, buy them raw to cook at home. If you are buying them already cooked, check for chemical preservatives.

• **Leavened whole grain bread:** slice it and store it in the fridge to make it last several days.

• **Seaweed:** are excellent nutrients that provide a lot with a small daily serving portion. The most recommended if you do not have much time are the arame and wakame (3 to 5 minutes of soaking) which can be added to almost any dish. The nori can be toasted lightly over a flame before putting it in salads or other dishes. At night, you can prepare a dessert for the following day: boil agar-agar and mix it with crushed fruit for a nutritious jelly.

• **Nuts and seeds:** provide good protein intake and can be eaten raw or lightly roasted. Combining seeds and legumes increases the protein value of the meal.

• **Wheat germ and brewer's yeast:** sprinkle in salads, stews, or grains and vegetables.

• **Plant-based protein:** in food stores there is a good assortment of plant-derived foods that perfectly replace meat and other animal protein, such as: tempeh, tofu, seitan and other food items such as soy burgers and sausages.

• **Sauerkraut:** Ideal to regenerate intestinal flora and alkalize the blood. It pairs well with soy sausages or veggie burgers.

• **Pureed vegetables or nuts:** from chickpeas, sesame seeds, sunflower seeds, walnuts, almonds, seaweed, etc. They can be used to enhance the flavors of soup and sauces or mix with salad dressing.

• **Good quality olive oil:** if possible, use extra virgin or, at least, virgin olive oil with low acidity.

• **Miso, sea salt, soy sauce, or tamari:** the salty and natural component that our palates need.

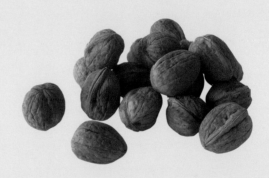

A BALANCED MENU

We should make sure we have enough carbohydrates, protein, fiber, vitamins, minerals, and some good fats. For instance:

• Start with a small raw vegetable salad.

• Choose a protein, a carbohydrate, and some cooked vegetables. This may be a single food like a stew (for instance lentils, rice, and vegetables) or combine a slice of grilled tofu with cooked grains, and cooked vegetables.

• Alternatively, if you have prepared soup, have that first and then follow, for example, with seitan steak grilled with salad or grains.

• For dessert, have a piece of fresh fruit, some applesauce, a few nuts (leave soaking at the beginning of the meal), or fruit jelly made from agar-agar.

We have at our disposal excellent products for healthy diets.

WHEN SHOULD FOOD BE PREPARED?

Let's take, for example, a full workday with a lunch break at noon, either in the same workplace or outside. There are certain foods that can be prepared the day before to combine as a meal.

For instance:

- Cooked whole grains such as rice, millet, bulgur wheat, quinoa, or couscous
- Noodles, whole wheat pasta
- Legumes such as lentils, chickpeas, or beans
- Hard boiled eggs
- Steamed vegetables such as green beans, squash, parsnips, and other vegetables
- Homemade tomato sauce
- Vegetable omelet (without potatoes)
- Corn on the cob (organic)
- Vegetable soups without potato
- Leafy greens that are washed, dried, and stored in an airtight container

DEPENDING ON WHERE YOU EAT

If you go home because you live close by, you can warm up hot foods and wash and chop vegetables for a salad. One trick to further save time is to have a few toppings ready in bottles, like mixed oil, vinegar, salt or soy sauce; just shake and add to your salad.

If the workplace has a kitchen or dining room, adapt the menu depending on what there is available (fridge, stove, etc.).

MEALS TO FIT YOUR NEEDS

Your daily activity has—or should have—much to do with your meals. So, your diet should be based on the amount of energy you use, whether it is more physical or intellectual work.

More about vegetables and fruits

- We recommend cleaning vegetables for salads, but do not cut or soak them because they lose vitamins. Before eating, they can be quickly chopped, either with a knife or mandolin, a device that cuts vegetables into strips or thin slices very quickly.
- Vegetables can be cooked the night before to eat them the next day, except potatoes, which ferment within a few hours.
- Another option is to make stir-fried vegetables, in which case we just need to cut them into thin slices or strips and put them in a lightly oiled pan and toss them until they are *al dente*, that is, halfway between raw and cooked. This takes no more than approximately 10 minutes between cutting and sautéing. Once done cooking, add pasta or cooked grains and a few seeds.
- Those with digestive problems should try to avoid fruit for dessert, though apparently the exception are apples and pears, as they are considered neutral fruits that do not interfere with the digestive process.
- If fruits are organically grown, it is better to eat them with their skin (where most of the vitamins and minerals are) after washing, but if they are conventionally grown, it is better to peel them because the chemicals used are on the outside.

FROZEN: YES OR NO?

Our recommendation is to always eat fresh, homemade, and natural foods; that is, unrefined and without chemical preservatives. However, if you like to cook you can prepare a few homemade patties using soy, rice, and vegetables (or other combinations) and keep in the freezer.

If you eat at home, take them out of the freezer in the morning before leaving for work. So, when you return at noon, just cook them on a griddle for a few minutes on each side. If there is a kitchen at work, bring them frozen in an airtight container and lunch will be ready to heat. The same applies for seitan (it takes a little more time, but it is easy) or vegetable stews.

USE THE STOVE, NOT THE MICROWAVE

Microwaves are too often used for heating food quickly. However, they are not recommended, since food undergoes drastic changes in their cell or protein structure. All food options given here can be heated in a lightly oiled pan in a few minutes.

PAY ATTENTION TO THE SEASONS

It is vital to try to be in harmony with nature and its seasonal changes. In cold weather we need more hot and comforting meals; whereas in warm weather, our food needs to refresh. Moreover, in spring and summer—if possible, and there is a green space nearby—it is best to make foods that can be eaten outside, such as a pasta salad, a salad with rice or other grains, a small vegetable omelet, seaweed and tofu, some fresh fruit or plain yogurt or kefir, and a few nuts.

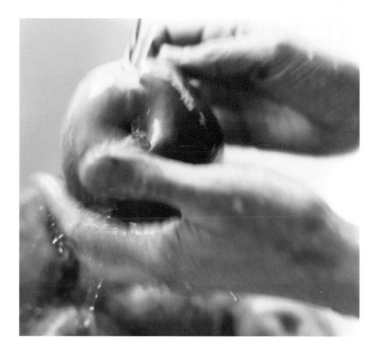

DRINKS

For those who are in the habit of drinking tea or coffee after eating, it is best to opt for healthier alternatives like green tea, chicory coffee, roasted grain drinks, rooibos tea, or red tea.

It is best to always eat fresh, natural foods.

Final note

All these recommendations will in one way or another, create positive changes in our body, which in turn will result in increased performance. There is nothing worse than eating poorly, quickly, or inadequately for you to spend the day feeling with low energy.

The important thing is to adopt healthy eating habits, even when you do not have a lot of time to eat. The secret is in choosing good foods and how you eat them.

The best diet in the world

- Mostly vegetable foods to avoid toxins in meat and fish
- Organic fruits, vegetables, seeds, and nuts that are naturally rich in micronutrients
- Unprocessed foods that are rich in fiber
- Low-protein products, such as tofu and tempeh
- Cooked vegetables and brown rice, to maximize nutritional content
- Vegetarian milk (soy, almond, rice)
- Freshly squeezed fruit juices
- Organic green tea, a powerful antioxidant
- Wild foods (vegetables, berries, seaweed, and mushrooms)
- Only fruits and vegetables that are in season
- Organic rice and whole wheat products; also all grains, even those less common in the West, like quinoa and millet
- Sesame seeds, pumpkin seeds, and sunflower for the brain and vitality
- Onion sprouts, lentils, and other seeds
- Oats and other grains for breakfast
- Brewer's yeast and wheat germ with fresh mixed salad
- Extra virgin olive oil
- Mineral water

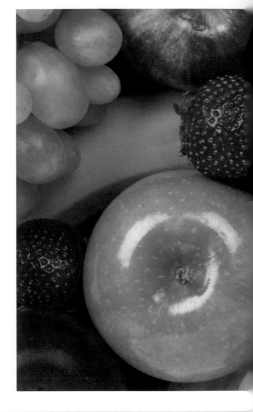

The worst diet in the world

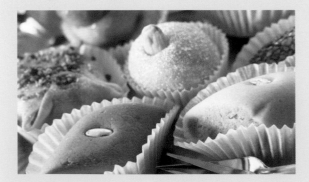

- Foods with high calorie count (more than the body is able to burn) that promote obesity
- Animal fats (beef, chicken with skin) that trigger cholesterol
- Meat artificially fattened with hormones and drugs
- Carbohydrates and simple sugars (refined flour and sugar, pastries, candy, chips, and soft drinks with sweeteners)
- Saturated fat in dairy products (cream, butter, fatty cheeses) and hydrogenated fats (margarine and vegetable shortening)

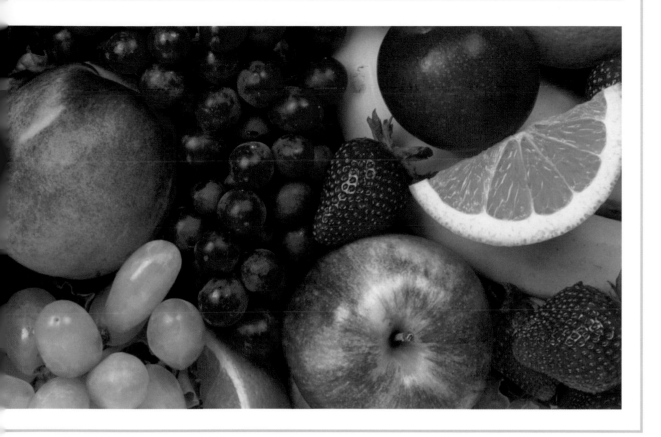

- Refined white sugar, an ingredient in a lot of prepackaged food
- Polyunsaturated vegetable oils that promote cancer and accelerate cellular aging
- Trans fats (vegetable oils and fats for frying)
- Cow's milk that leads to allergies and autoimmune disorders
- Lack of micronutrients, particularly low intake of fresh fruit and vegetables
- Pre-fried potatoes and refined flour
- Canned fruits in syrup
- Iceberg lettuce and strawberries grown with the use of pesticides
- Tomato sauce, rich in sugar and sodium
- Low intake of fiber, minerals, and fresh vitamins
- Unpurified tap water that contains lead and other heavy metals
- Three or four coffees a day, especially dark roast
- Daily intake of alcohol (especially white drinks with added sugar) and cigarettes
- Fast food

Recipes

GLOSSARY

FOOD	SOURCE OF . . .	GOOD FOR . . .
Chicory	Folic acid, potassium, iron, vitamins A and C	Before and after pregnancy. Purifying, detoxifying and gently diuretic and liver stimulant.
Avocado	Potassium, vitamin E and A, essential fatty acids	Heart, blood circulation, and skin. Relieves PMS symptoms and protects against cancer.
Garlic	Sulfates, antibacterial, and fungicidal	Protects against heart disease, reduces cholesterol and hypertension. Combats fungi and bacteria.
Apricot	Beta-carotene, potassium, iron, soluble fiber	Skin and circulatory disorders. Protects against cancer. Dry, it treats constipation and high blood pressure.
Artichoke	Phosphorus, iron	Digestion because it stimulates the liver and gallbladder. Treats gout, arthritis, and rheumatism.
Beans	Protein, carbohydrates, fiber, B vitamins, minerals, folic acid, selenium, iron, zinc	Heart health and circulatory system. Mitigate hypertension and reduce cholesterol. Prevent cancer and regulate bowel function.
Blueberry	Vitamin C	Treatment and prevention of cystitis. Prevents cancer and boosts the immune system.
Brown rice	B vitamins, proteins	Celiac, since it contains no gluten. Good treatment for diarrhea. Boosts energy.
Oats	Calcium, potassium, magnesium, vitamins B and E	Reduces cholesterol and hypertension. Prevents cancer and cardiovascular disease.
Sweet potato	Vitamins C and E, beta-carotene and other carotenoids, proteins	Eye problems. Skincare and prevents cancer.

FOOD	SOURCE OF . . .	GOOD FOR . . .
Broccoli	Vitamins A and C, folic acid, riboflavin, potassium, iron	Anemia, chronic fatigue, before and during pregnancy, skin problems. Protects against cancer.
Alfalfa sprouts	Vitamins A, B, C, E and K, calcium	The nervous system, bones, and skin.
Squash	Vitamins A, B and C, folic acid, potassium	Protects against cancer and mitigates respiratory diseases. Skincare.
Thistle	Vitamins A and C, iron, calcium, phosphorus, carotenes	Prevents eye conditions such as macular degeneration. It also protects against cancer and for anemia.
Chestnut	Fiber, vitamins E and B6, potassium	Easily digestible. Suitable for making flour in case of gluten intolerance. Boosts energy.
Brazil nuts	Protein, selenium, vitamin E and B	One of the richest sources of selenium, an essential mineral that protects against cardiovascular disease and prostate cancer.
Onion	Vitamin C, sulfate compounds	Prevents blood clots, lowers cholesterol, fights bronchitis, asthma, chest infections, gout, and arthritis.
Cherry	Vitamin C, potassium, magnesium, flavonoids	Boosts immune system, alleviates arthritis, and rheumatism. Protects against cancer and relieves gout.
Mushroom	Vitamin B12, vitamin E, zinc, proteins	Depression, anxiety, and fatigue.
Chili	Vitamin C, carotenoids, capsaicin	Circulation and digestion. Fights lung diseases and stomach infections.

GLOSSARY

FOOD	SOURCE OF . . .	GOOD FOR . . .
Parsnip	Vitamins B and E, potassium, folic acid	Pregnancy, and against fatigue, colds, and diabetes.
Plum	Vitamins C and E, beta-carotene, malic acid	The heart, circulation, and digestion. Relieves fluid retention.
Cabbage	Vitamins A, C, and E, folic acid	Prevents cancer, stomach ulcer, lung infections, skin diseases, and anemia.
Kale	Beta-carotene, vitamin C, phosphorus, sulfur, iron, potassium, calcium, folic acid	Boosts immune system and prevents cancer. Care of the skin and eyes.
Brussels sprouts	Vitamin C and beta-carotene	Protect against cancer and skin conditions.
Cauliflower	Vitamin C, folic acid, sulfur	Prevents cancer and boosts immune system.
Coriander	Flavonoids, linalol	Digestion. Relieves flatulence and intestinal disorders. Recommended against stress.
Asparagus	Vitamin C, riboflavin, folic acid, potassium, phosphorus	Diuretic, recommended against cystitis and fluid retention. Suitable for rheumatism and arthritis, but not for gout.
Spinach	Chlorophyll, folic acid, beta-carotene, iron	Skin and eye care, and during pregnancy.Protect against cancer.
Raspberry	Vitamin C, calcium, potassium, magnesium, iron, soluble fiber	The immune system. Prevents cancer and relieves mouth ulcers.
Strawberry	Vitamins C and E, beta-carotene, soluble fiber	Combat arthritis, gout, liver disorders, and anemia. Prevents cancer.
Peas	Beta-carotene, folic acid, thiamin, vitamin C, protein	Combat digestive problems, stress, and tension.
Fig	Beta-carotene, iron, potassium, fiber	Boosts energy. Relieves constipation and digestive disorders. Combat anemia and prevents cancer.

FOOD	SOURCE OF . . .	GOOD FOR . . .
Dandelion leaves	Beta-carotene, carotenoids, iron	Relieves fluid retention, liver disorders, and PMS.
Eggs	Protein, vitamins A, B12, D, and E, iron, lecithin, zinc	Prevent cancer and cardiovascular disease. Recommended against anemia and rheumatoid arthritis. Enhance sexual stamina in men.
Ginger	Circulation stimulating compounds	Post operation, circulation, fever, and cough.
Green beans	Vitamin A and C, potassium, folic acid	Skin, hair, and digestive problems.
Kiwi	Vitamin C, beta-carotene, potassium, bioflavonoids, fiber	The immune system and skin. Relieves colds and digestive disorders.
Milk	Calcium, zinc, riboflavin, proteins	Stimulates growth and strengthens bones. Suitable for convalescence.
Lettuce	Vitamins A and C, folic acid, potassium, calcium, phosphorus	Combat insomnia and stress. Recommended for bronchitis.
Lime	Vitamin C, bioflavonoids, potassium	The immune system. Relieves flu, coughs, and colds. Protects against cancer.
Lemon	Vitamin C, bioflavonoids, potassium	The immune system and digestion. Mitigates mouth ulcers and gum disease.
Sweet corn	Fiber, protein, folic acid, vitamins A and E	Provides fiber. Boosts energy.
Mango	Vitamin C, beta-carotene, potassium, flavonoids	Skin disorders and convalescence. Boosts immune system and prevents cancer.
Apple	Carotenes, pectin, vitamin C, potassium	The immune system, digestion, heart, and circulation. Recommended against colds, diarrhea, and cholesterol.

Glossary

GLOSSARY

FOOD	SOURCE OF . . .	GOOD FOR . . .
Peach	Beta-carotene, vitamin C, potassium, flavonoids	Pregnancy and as a laxative. Recommended for reducing cholesterol and for low salt diets.
Cantaloupe	Vitamins A, B and C, potassium, folic acid	Arthritis, gout, mild colds, and urinary problems.
Mint	Flavonoid, menthol, antispasmodic essential oils	Cases of indigestion, gastritis, inflammation, and gas. Apply it to the temples to relieve migraines.
Bilberry	Vitamin C, carotenoids	See blackberry
Blackberry	Vitamins E and C, potassium, fiber	The heart, circulation, and skin. Also a good cancer preventative.
Turnip	Vitamins A and C, minerals	Combat skin problems and prevents cancer.
Orange and tangerine	Vitamins C and B6, potassium, thiamine, folic acid, calcium, iron, bioflavonoids	The defenses and heart. Mitigate infections and hypertension. The skin and cardiovascular system.
Olive	Monounsaturated oil, antioxidants, vitamin E	Everyone, except those with gluten intolerance. Combat stress and prevents constipation. Relieves hemorrhoids.
Bread	Fiber, iron, vitamins B and E, proteins	Fight hypertension, fatigue, and colds. Prevent cancer.
Raisins	Vitamin B6, niacin, beta-carotene, potassium, iron, fiber	Growth and immune system. Helps mitigate anemia, fatigue, and digestive problems.
Potato	Vitamins B and C, fiber and minerals	Skin and eyes. In the form of juice, mitigates fever.
Cucumber	Beta-carotene (skin), silicon, potassium, folic acid	

FOOD	SOURCE OF . . .	GOOD FOR . . .
Pear	Vitamin C, soluble fiber	Reduce convalescence and cholesterol. Energy.
Parsley	Vitamins A and C, iron, calcium, potassium	Relieves fluid retention, PMS, gout, rheumatism, and anemia. Diuretic and anti-inflammatory.
Pepper	Vitamin C, folic acid, beta-carotene, potassium	Skin and mucous membrane disorders. Boosts the immune system. Improves night vision and color.
Pineapple	Vitamin C, enzymes	Relieves angina, arthritis, fever, chills, sore throat.
Banana	Potassium, fiber, magnesium, vitamin A, folic acid	Prevents muscle cramps. Excellent for digestion and against chronic fatigue syndrome.
Grapefruit	Vitamin C, beta-carotene, potassium, bioflavonoids	Boosts immune system, mitigates circulatory problems, sore throats, and bleeding gums.
Leek	Vitamins A and C, folic acid, iron, potassium	Lung and voice disorders, especially sore throat. Combat hypertension and excess cholesterol.
Cheese	Protein, calcium and vitamin B12, zinc	Bones, teeth, and the prevention/ treatment of osteoporosis.
Radish	Vitamin C, magnesium, iron, sulfur, potassium	The liver and bladder. Prevents cancer and relieves indigestion and respiratory problems.
Rhubarb	Calcium, potassium, manganese, vitamins A and C	Relieves colds.
Seeds and nuts	Unsaturated fats, proteins, zinc, selenium, fiber	Fertility and sexual vigor. Fight diabetes, colds and varicose veins. Promote intellectual functions.

GLOSSARY

FOOD	SOURCE OF . . .	GOOD FOR . . .
Green Tea	Powerful antioxidants, vitamins E and K	Youthfulness, heart health, and prevent cancer. Combat fatigue.
Tofu and other soy products	Protein and genistein	Vegetarians and diabetics. Milk intolerance. Protects against breast cancer and prostate cancer.
Tomato	Beta carotene, lycopene, vitamins C and E, potassium	Heart health and fertility. Prevents cancer and relieves skin disorders.
Wheat and whole wheat flour	Fiber, vitamins B and E, magnesium, zinc, and selenium	Source of vitality and essential nutrients.
Grape	Vitamin C, natural sugars, flavonoids	Anemia, fatigue and convalescence. Prevents cancer and helps to regain weight.
Yogurt	Calcium, zinc, riboflavin, proteins, good bacteria	Immune system. Relieves diarrhea and cystitis. Recommended for preventing and treating osteoporosis.
Carrot	Vitamin A, carotenoids, folic acid, potassium, magnesium	Eyesight and circulation. Prevents cardiovascular disease and cancer. Also good for skincare and mucous membranes.

FIVE STAR SUPERFOODS

Fruit

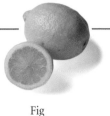

Avocado		Lemon	Pear
Apricot		Apple	Pineapple
Blueberry		Cantaloupe	Banana
Date		Blackberry	Grapefruit
Raspberry	Fig	Orange	Watermelon
Strawberry	Kiwi	Papaya	Grape

Vegetables

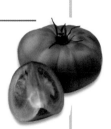

Chicory	Squash	Red cabbage	Potato
Artichoke	Thistle	Green cabbage	Peppers
Alfalfa	Onion	Asparagus	Leek
Celery	Mushroom	Spinach	Radish
Sweet potato	Sauerkraut	Turnip	Tomato
Broccoli	Kale	Nettle	Carrot

Whole Grains   Nuts, legumes, seeds, and sprouts

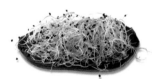

Buckwheat	Almond	Walnut
Rice	Cashew	Pumpkin seeds
Oats	Hazelnut	Sunflower seeds
Barley	Sprouts	Sesame seeds
Millet	Lentil	Soybeans and soy products:
Wheat and wheat germ	Peanut butter	tofu, tempeh (and lecithin)

Dairy   Spices, herbs, and medicinal plants

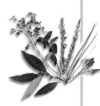

Kefir	Garlic	Fenugreek	Parsley
Goat milk	Caraway	Ginkgo Biloba	Rosemary
Natural yogurt and bifidus	Cinnamon	Ginger	Green tea
Cottage cheese	Dandelion	Mint	Thyme

Other

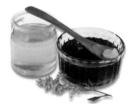

Oils: sunflower, walnut, grapeseed, etc.	Aloe vera	Horseradish
	Echinacea	Licorice
Extra virgin olive oil	Royal jelly	Maple syrup
Mineral water	Beet yeast	Antioxidant supplements
Algae and spirulina	Molasses	Dietary supplements
	Honey, pollen, propolis	Fruit and vegetable juices

LEARN MORE—BIBLIOGRAPHY

Nutrition

Salud y nutrición. Recetas nutritivas que curan. *Dr. James F. Balch y Phyllis A. Balch.* Ed. Océano Ambar, Barcelona, 2004

The New Whole Foods Encyclopedia. *Rebecca Wood.* Penguin, N. York, 1999

The Healing Nutrients Within *Dr. Eric R. Braverman.* Keats, New Cannan, 1987

La alternativa vegetariana. *Vic Sussman.* Integral, Barcelona, 1992

Cuerpo radiante. *Dr. Bernard Jensen.* Ed. Océano Ambar, Barcelona, 2002

Vinagre de sidra. *Marie-France Muller.* Ed. Océano Ambar, Barcelona, 2002

Adelgazar es natural. *Adriana Ortemberg.* Ed. Océano Ambar, Barcelona, 2001

Antioxidantes para rejuvenecer. *Adriana Ortemberg.* Ed. Océano Ambar, Barcelona, 2001

Suplementos energéticos. Guía práctica de suplementos dietéticos. *Earl Mindell.* Ed. Océano Ambar, Barcelona, 2002

El poder curativo de los alimentos. *Vicki Edgson & Ian Marber.* Ed. Parramon, Barcelona, 2001

La gran guía de la composición de los alimentos. *Dr. Ibrahim Elmadfa.* Integral, Barcelona, 1989, 1996

Alimentos saludables. *Amanda Ursell.* Ed. Raíces, Madrid, 2002

Los alimentos más sanos. *Manolo Núñez y Claudina Navarro.* Cuerpomente, Barcelona, 2001

Alimentos, medicina milagrosa. *Jean Carper.* Amat, Barcelona, 2000

La Biblia de la nutrición óptima. *Patrick Holford.* Robinbook, Barcelona, 1999

En la cama con el Doctor Comida. *Vicki Edgson e Ian Marber.* Ed. Océano Ambar, Barcelona, 2003

La combinación de los alimentos. *Herbert M. Shelton.* Obelisco, Barcelona, 1996

Las claves de la nutrición. *Désiré Mérien.* Ed. Ibis, Barcelona, 1995

Guía de la salud natural Bircher. *R. Kunz Bircher.* Martínez Roca, Barcelona, 1994

La cura de la savia y el zumo de limón. *K. A. Beyer.* Obelisco, Barcelona, 1990

El Tao de la nutrición. *Dr. Maoshing Ni.* Ed. Océano Ambar, Barcelona, 2003

Élever son enfant . . . autrement. *Catherine Dumonteil-Kremer.* La Plage ed., Sète, 2003

Los mejores alimentos para los niños. *Michael van Straten y Barbara Griggs.* Blume, Barcelona, 2001

Alimentación infantil natural. *Paloma Zamora.* Integral, Barcelona 1992

Alimentación natural infantil. *Vicki Edgson.* Ed. Océano Ambar, Barcelona, 2004

¿Sabemos comer? *Dr. Andrew Weil.* Ed. Urano, Barcelona, 2001

Koch Zeit. Cocina rápida y sana con 4 ingredientes. *Alexander Herrmann.* Zabert Sandmann, Munich, 2000

Enzyme Therapy. *Dr. Anthony Cichoke.* Avery, N. York, 1999

Alimentación natural. *VV. AA.* Cuerpomente, Barcelona, 2002

¡Salve su cuerpo! *Dra. C. Kousmine.* Ed. Javier Vergara, Buenos Aires, 1993

La alimentación equilibrada. *Dr. Barnet Meltzer.* Ed. Océano Ambar, Barcelona, 2003

Vivir sin acidez. *Norbert Treutwein.* Ed. Océano Ambar, Barcelona, 2004

Comida para vivir feliz. *Klaus Oberweil.* Ed. Océano Ambar, Barcelona, 2004

Técnicas culinarias. Técnicas y estilos de cocción y preparación de los alimentos. *VV. AA.* Ed. Océano Ambar, Barcelona, 2004

El gourmet vegetariano. *Colin Spencer.* Integral, Barcelona, 1992

Picture Perfect Weight Loss. *Dr. Howard M. Shapiro.* Rodale, London, 2004

Organic Superfoods. *Michael van Straten.* Mitchell Beazley, London, 1999

Food & Soul. *Brahma Kumaris.* Health Com, Deerfield Beach, 2001

Ingredients

El huerto familiar ecológico. *Mariano Bueno.* Integral RBA, Barcelona, 1999

El huerto biológico. *Claude Aubert.* Integral, Barcelona, 1985

El libro de la pasta y la pizza. *Iona Purtí.* Integral, Barcelona, 1996

Aloe Vera. *Shia Green.* Ed. Océano Ambar, Barcelona, 2001

Tempeh, la mejor proteína vegetal. *Shia Green.* Ed. Océano Ambar, Barcelona, 2002

Rooibos. *Jörg Zittlau.* Ed. Océano Ambar, Barcelona, 2002

Algas, las verduras del mar. *Montse Bradford.* Ed. Océano Ambar, Barcelona, 3rd ed., 2003

Germinados. *Luisa Martín Rueda.* Ed. Océano Ambar, Barcelona, 2001

Hierba del Trigo. *Ann Wigmore.* Ed. Océano Ambar, Barcelona, 1999

Té verde. *Iona Purtí & A. Marcelo Pascual.* Ed. Océano Ambar, Barcelona, 2nd ed., 2003

Ginkgo Biloba. *Dr. M. Pros.* Ed. Océano Ambar, Barcelona, 2000

El libro del yogur. *Iona Purtí, Jaume Rosselló.* Integral, Barcelona, 1995

El libro del tofu. *Iona Purtí.* Ed. Océano Ambar, Barcelona, 2nd ed., 2003

Kéfir, un «yogur» para rejuvenecer. *Mercedes Blasco.* Ed. Océano Ambar, Barcelona, 2nd ed., 2003

Especias y plantas aromáticas. *Dr. J. L Berdonces.* Ed. Océano Ambar, Barcelona, 2001

Natural Cooking

Natural Foods Cookbook. *Charles Gerrras,* ed. Rodale Press, Emmaus, 1984

Cocine con poca grasa. *Jenni Muir.* Reader's Digest, Mexico, 2000

El libro de la cocina natural. *Iona Purtí, Jaume Rosselló, Josan Ruiz.* Integral, Barcelona, 6th ed. 1998

Cocina natural. *Claude Aubert y Emmanuelle Aubert.* Ed. Océano Ámbar, Barcelona, 1995

La nueva cocina energética. *Montse Bradford.* Ed. Océano Ambar, Barcelona, 6th ed., 2004

Alquimia en la cocina (La nueva cocina energética—segunda parte). *Montse Bradford.* Ed. Océano Ambar, Barcelona, 2004

El libro de las proteínas vegetales. *Montse Bradford.* Ed. Océano Ambar, Barcelona, 2ª ed., 2004

Aperitivos y platos ligeros combinados. *Hilda Parisi.* Ed. Océano Ambar, Barcelona, 2004

Cocina rápida vegetariana. *Adriana Ortemberg.* Ed. Océano Ambar, Barcelona, 2ª ed., 2003

Desayunos naturales. *Mercedes Blasco.* Ed. Océano Ambar, Barcelona, 2ª ed., 2004

Cocinar. . . ¡a todo vapor! *Hilda Parisi.* Ed. Océano Ambar, Barcelona, 2ª ed., 2003

Superzumos. *Rodolfo Román & Claudia Antist.* Ed. Océano Ambar, Barcelona, 2004

Cocina Feng Shui de los 5 elementos. *Iona Purtí & Adriana Ortemberg.* Ed. Océano Ambar, Barcelona, 2003

Ensaladas. *Adriana Ortemberg.* Ed. Océano Ambar, Barcelona, 2003

Yoga y cocina. *Centro Sivananda Vedanta.* Integral RBA, Barcelona, 1999

Sopas Bar. *Claudia Antist.* Ed. Océano Ambar, Barcelona, 2003

Desserts Bio. *Valérie Cupillard.* La Plage ed., Sète, 2003

Ancient Secret of the Fountain of Youth Cookbook. *Devanando Otfried Weise.* Harbor, Gig Harbor, 1998

My Food Diary

My Food Diary

My Food Diary

_____

_____

_____

_____

_____

_____

_____

_____

_____

_____

_____

_____

_____

_____

_____

_____

_____

_____

_____